Psychoradiology

Editor

QIYONG GONG

NEUROIMAGING CLINICS OF NORTH AMERICA

www.neuroimaging.theclinics.com

Consulting Editor
SURESH K. MUKHERJI

February 2020 • Volume 30 • Number 1

ELSEVIER

1600 John F. Kennedy Boulevard ● Suite 1800 ● Philadelphia, Pennsylvania, 19103-2899

http://www.neuroimaging.theclinics.com

NEUROIMAGING CLINICS OF NORTH AMERICA Volume 30, Number 1
February 2020 ISSN 1052-5149, ISBN 13: 978-0-323-70886-9

Editor: John Vassallo (j.vassallo@elsevier.com)
Developmental Editor: Casey Potter

Neuroimaging Clinics of North America (ISSN 1052-5149) is published quarterly by Elsevier Inc., 360 Park Avenue South, New York, NY 10010-1710. Months of issue are February, May, August, and November. Business and editorial offices: 1600 John F. Kennedy Blvd., Suite 1800, Philadelphia, PA 19103-2899. Business and editorial offices: 6277 Sea Harbor Drive, Orlando, FL 32887-4800. Periodicals postage paid at New York, NY, and additional mailing offices. Subscription prices are USD 397 per year for US individuals, USD 686 per year for US institutions, USD 100 per year for US students and residents, USD 451 per year for Canadian individuals, USD 874 per year for Canadian institutions, USD 541 per year for international individuals, USD 874 per year for international institutions, USD 100 per year for Canadian students and residents and USD 260 per year for foreign students and residents. To receive student/resident rate, orders must be accompanied by name of affiliated institution, date of term, and the *signature* of program/residency coordinator on institution letterhead. Orders will be billed at individual rate until proof of status is received. Foreign air speed delivery is included in all *Clinics* subscription prices. All prices are subject to change without notice. POSTMASTER: Send address changes to *Neuroimaging Clinics of North America*, Elsevier Health Sciences Division, Subscription **Customer Service, 3251 Riverport Lane, Maryland Heights, MO 63043. Telephone: 1-800-654-2452 (U.S. and Canada); 314-447-8871 (outside U.S. and Canada). Fax: 314-447-8029. E-mail: journalscustomerservice-usa@elsevier.com (for print support); journalsonlinesupport-usa@elsevier.com (for online support).**

Reprints. For copies of 100 or more of articles in this publication, please contact the Commercial Reprints Department, Elsevier Inc., 360 Park Avenue South, New York, NY 10010-1710. Tel.: 212-633-3874; Fax: 212-633-3820; E-mail: reprints@elsevier.com.

Neuroimaging Clinics of North America is covered by *Excerpta Medical/EMBASE,* the RSNA Index of Imaging Literature, *MEDLINE/PubMed (Index Medicus),* MEDLINE/MEDLARS, SciSearch, Research Alert, and Neuroscience Citation Index.

PROGRAM OBJECTIVE
The goal of *Neuroimaging Clinics of North America* is to keep practicing radiologists and radiology residents up to date with current clinical practice in radiology by providing timely articles reviewing the state of the art in patient care.

TARGET AUDIENCE
Practicing radiologists, radiology residents, and other healthcare professionals who utilize neuroimaging findings to provide patient care.

LEARNING OBJECTIVES
Upon completion of this activity, participants will be able to:
1. Review major psychiatric imaging methods, including resting state fMRI and MR spectroscopy, as well as image analysis protocols for psychiatry.
2. Discuss general issues related to subtyping heterogeneous psychiatric syndromes, as well as monitoring and predicting treatment response using psychoradiological biomarkers for psychopharmaceutical effects.
3. Recognize current clinical applications of psychiatric imaging relevant to common psychiatric disorders including schizophrenia, major depression, bipolar disorder, autism spectrum disorder and attention deficit hyperactivity disorder.

ACCREDITATION
The Elsevier Office of Continuing Medical Education (EOCME) is accredited by the Accreditation Council for Continuing Medical Education (ACCME) to provide continuing medical education for physicians.

The EOCME designates this journal-based CME activity for a maximum of 11 *AMA PRA Category 1 Credit*(s)™. Physicians should claim only the credit commensurate with the extent of their participation in the activity.

All other healthcare professionals requesting continuing education credit for this enduring material will be issued a certificate of participation.

DISCLOSURE OF CONFLICTS OF INTEREST
The EOCME assesses conflict of interest with its instructors, faculty, planners, and other individuals who are in a position to control the content of CME activities. All relevant conflicts of interest that are identified are thoroughly vetted by EOCME for fair balance, scientific objectivity, and patient care recommendations. EOCME is committed to providing its learners with CME activities that promote improvements or quality in healthcare and not a specific proprietary business or a commercial interest.

The planning committee, staff, authors and editors listed below have identified no financial relationships or relationships to products or devices they or their spouse/life partner have with commercial interest related to the content of this CME activity:
Osamu Abe, MD, PhD; Azeezat Azeez, PhD; Bharat B. Biswal, PhD; Stefan Borgwardt, MD; Donna Y. Chen, BE; Kai Chen, PhD; Guusje Collin, PhD; Louisa Dahmani, PhD; Christos Davatzikos, PhD; Yong Fan, PhD; Cynthia H.Y. Fu, MD, PhD; Jessica B. Girault, PhD; Qiyong Gong, MD, PhD; Synthia Guimond, PhD; Elena I. Ivleva, MD, PhD; Kouhei Kamiya, MD, PhD; Sinead Kelly, PhD; Alison Kemp; Matcheri S. Keshavan, MD; Pradeep Kuttysankaran; Fei Li, MD, PhD; Hesheng Liu, PhD; William J. Liu, BSc; Paulo Lizano, MD, PhD; Su Lui, MD, PhD; Suresh K. Mukherji, MD, MBA, FACR; Joseph Piven, MD; John D. Port, MD, PhD; Casey Potter; Konasale M. Prasad, MD; Liesbeth Reneman, MD, PhD; Henricus Gerardus Ruhé, MD, PhD; André Schmidt, PhD; Anouk Schrantee, PhD; John A. Sweeney, PhD; Halide B. Turkozer, MD; John Vassallo; Danhong Wang, MD, PhD; Dongsheng Wu, MD.

UNAPPROVED/OFF-LABEL USE DISCLOSURE
The EOCME requires CME faculty to disclose to the participants:
1. When products or procedures being discussed are off-label, unlabelled, experimental, and/or investigational (not US Food and Drug Administration [FDA] approved); and
2. Any limitations on the information presented, such as data that are preliminary or that represent ongoing research, interim analyses, and/or unsupported opinions. Faculty may discuss information about pharmaceutical agents that is outside of FDA-approved labelling. This information is intended solely for CME and is not intended to promote off-label use of these medications. If you have any questions, contact the medical affairs department of the manufacturer for the most recent prescribing information.

TO ENROLL
To enroll in the *Neuroimaging Clinics of North America* Continuing Medical Education program, call customer service at 1-800-654-2452 or sign up online at http://www.theclinics.com/home/cme. The CME program is available to subscribers for an additional annual fee of USD 245.

METHOD OF PARTICIPATION
In order to claim credit, participants must complete the following:
1. Complete enrolment as indicated above.
2. Read the activity.

3. Complete the CME Test and Evaluation. Participants must achieve a score of 70% on the test. All CME Tests and Evaluations must be completed online.

CME INQUIRIES/SPECIAL NEEDS

For all CME inquiries or special needs, please contact elsevierCME@elsevier.com.

NEUROIMAGING CLINICS OF NORTH AMERICA

SERIES OF RELATED INTEREST

MRI Clinics of North America
Mri.theclinics.com
PET Clinics
pet.theclinics.com
Radiologic Clinics of North America
Radiologic.theclinics.com

THE CLINICS ARE AVAILABLE ONLINE!
Access your subscription at:
www.theclinics.com

Contributors

CONSULTING EDITOR

SURESH K. MUKHERJI, MD, MBA, FACR
Clinical Professor, Marian University, Director
of Head and Neck Radiology, ProScan
Imaging, Regional Medical Director, Envision
Physician Services, Carmel, Indiana, USA

EDITOR

QIYONG GONG, MD, PhD
Clinical Professor of Radiology, Director of
Huaxi MR Research Center (HMRRC), Section
of Neuroradiology, Department of Radiology,
West China Hospital of Sichuan University,
Chengdu, Sichuan Province, China; President,
Shenjing Hospital of China Medical University,
Shenyang, Liaoning Province, China;
Associate Editor, *American Journal of
Psychiatry*

AUTHORS

OSAMU ABE, MD, PhD
Department of Radiology, University of Tokyo,
Tokyo, Japan

AZEEZAT AZEEZ, PhD
Department of Biomedical Engineering, New
Jersey Institute of Technology, Newark, New
Jersey, USA

BHARAT B. BISWAL, PhD
The Clinical Hospital of Chengdu Brain Science
Institute, MOE Key Laboratory for
Neuroinformation, Center for Information in
Medicine, School of Life Science and
Technology, University of Electronic Science
and Technology of China, Chengdu, China;
Department of Biomedical Engineering, New
Jersey Institute of Technology, Newark, New
Jersey, USA

STEFAN BORGWARDT, MD
Department of Psychiatry (UPK), University of
Basel, Basel, Switzerland; Department of

Psychiatry and Psychotherapy, University of
Lübeck, Lübeck, Germany

DONNA Y. CHEN, BE
Department of Biomedical Engineering, New
Jersey Institute of Technology, Newark, New
Jersey, USA

KAI CHEN, PhD
The Clinical Hospital of Chengdu Brain Science
Institute, MOE Key Laboratory for
Neuroinformation, Center for Information in
Medicine, School of Life Science and
Technology, University of Electronic
Science and Technology of China, Chengdu,
China

GUUSJE COLLIN, PhD
Research Affiliate, McGovern Institute for Brain
Research, Massachusetts Institute of
Technology, Cambridge, Massachusetts, USA;
University Medical Center Utrecht Brain
Center, Utrecht, The Netherlands

LOUISA DAHMANI, PhD
Research Fellow, Athinoula A. Martinos Center for Biomedical Imaging, Department of Radiology, Massachusetts General Hospital, Harvard Medical School, Charlestown, Massachusetts, USA

CHRISTOS DAVATZIKOS, PhD
Professor, Center for Biomedical Image Computing and Analytics, Department of Radiology, Perelman School of Medicine, University of Pennsylvania, Philadelphia, Pennsylvania, USA

YONG FAN, PhD
Center for Biomedical Image Computing and Analytics, Department of Radiology, Perelman School of Medicine, University of Pennsylvania, Philadelphia, Pennsylvania, USA

CYNTHIA H.Y. FU, MD, PhD
Professor, School of Psychology, University of East London, Centre for Affective Disorders, Institute of Psychiatry, Psychology and Neuroscience, King's College London, London, United Kingdom

JESSICA B. GIRAULT, PhD
Carolina Institute for Developmental Disabilities, The University of North Carolina at Chapel Hill School of Medicine, Chapel Hill, North Carolina, USA

QIYONG GONG, MD, PhD
Clinical Professor of Radiology, Director of Huaxi MR Research Center (HMRRC), Section of Neuroradiology, Department of Radiology, West China Hospital of Sichuan University, Chengdu, Sichuan Province, China; President, Shenjing Hospital of China Medical University, Shenyang, Liaoning Province, China; Associate Editor, *American Journal of Psychiatry*

SYNTHIA GUIMOND, PhD
Scientist, Assistant Professor, Department of Psychiatry, The Royal's Institute of Mental Health Research, University of Ottawa, Ottawa, Canada

ELENA I. IVLEVA, MD, PhD
Department of Psychiatry, The University of Texas Southwestern Medical Center, Dallas, Texas, USA

KOUHEI KAMIYA, MD, PhD
Department of Radiology, University of Tokyo, Tokyo, Japan

SINEAD KELLY, PhD
Instructor of Psychiatry, Beth Israel Deaconess Medical Center, Harvard Medical School, Boston, Massachusetts, USA

MATCHERI S. KESHAVAN, MD
Stanley Cobb Professor and Academic Chair for Psychiatry, Department of Psychiatry, Beth Israel Deaconess Medical Center, Harvard Medical School, Boston, Massachusetts, USA

FEI LI, MD, PhD
Huaxi MR Research Center (HMRRC), Department of Radiology, West China Hospital of Sichuan University, Psychoradiology Research Unit of Chinese Academy of Medical Sciences, West China Hospital of Sichuan University, Chengdu, China

HESHENG LIU, PhD
Associate Professor, Athinoula A. Martinos Center for Biomedical Imaging, Department of Radiology, Massachusetts General Hospital, Harvard Medical School, Charlestown, Massachusetts, USA

WILLIAM J. LIU, BSc
Undergraduate Student, Department of Neuroscience, Grossman Institute of Neurobiology, The College, The University of Chicago, Chicago, Illinois, USA

PAULO LIZANO, MD, PhD
Instructor of Psychiatry, Beth Israel Deaconess Medical Center, Harvard Medical School, Boston, Massachusetts, USA

SU LUI, MD, PhD
Huaxi MR Research Center (HMRRC), Department of Radiology, West China Hospital of Sichuan University, Psychoradiology Research Unit of Chinese Academy of Medical Sciences, West China Hospital of Sichuan University, Chengdu, China

JOSEPH PIVEN, MD
Carolina Institute for Developmental Disabilities, The University of North Carolina at Chapel Hill School of Medicine, Chapel Hill, North Carolina, USA

JOHN D. PORT, MD, PhD
Professor, Department of Radiology,
Associate Professor, Department of
Psychiatry, Mayo Clinic, Rochester,
Minnesota, USA

KONASALE M. PRASAD, MD
Associate Professor of Psychiatry and
Bioengineering, University of Pittsburgh School
of Medicine, Swanson School of Engineering,
University of Pittsburgh, Veterans Affairs
Pittsburgh Healthcare System, Pittsburgh,
Pennsylvania, USA

LIESBETH RENEMAN, MD, PhD
Department of Radiology and Nuclear
Medicine, Professor and Neuroradiologist,
Amsterdam UMC, Academic Medical Center,
Amsterdam, The Netherlands

HENRICUS GERARDUS RUHÉ, MD, PhD
Associate Professor and Psychiatrist,
Department of Psychiatry, Radboud University
Medical Centre, Donders Institute for Brain,
Cognition and Behavior, Radboud University,
Nijmegen, The Netherlands

ANDRÉ SCHMIDT, PhD
Department of Psychiatry (UPK), University of
Basel, Basel, Switzerland

ANOUK SCHRANTEE, PhD
Department of Radiology and Nuclear
Medicine, Assistant Professor, Amsterdam
UMC, Academic Medical Center, Amsterdam,
The Netherlands

JOHN A. SWEENEY, PhD
Department of Psychiatry and Behavioral
Neuroscience, University of Cincinnati,
Cincinnati, Ohio, USA

HALIDE B. TURKOZER, MD
Department of Psychiatry, The University of
Texas Southwestern Medical Center, Dallas,
Texas, USA

DANHONG WANG, MD, PhD
Assistant Professor, Athinoula A. Martinos
Center for Biomedical Imaging, Department of
Radiology, Massachusetts General Hospital,
Harvard Medical School, Charlestown,
Massachusetts, USA

DONGSHENG WU, MD
Huaxi MR Research Center (HMRRC),
Department of Radiology, West China Hospital
of Sichuan University, Psychoradiology
Research Unit of Chinese Academy of Medical
Sciences, West China Hospital of Sichuan
University, Chengdu, China

Contents

Psychoradiology is an emerging discipline at the intersection between radiology and psychiatry. It holds promise for playing a role in clinical diagnosis, evaluation of treatment response and prognosis, and illness risk prediction for patients with psychiatric disorders. Addressing complex issues, such as the biological heterogeneity of psychiatric syndromes and unclear neurobiological mechanisms underpinning radiological abnormalities, is a challenge that needs to be resolved. With the advance of multimodal imaging and more efforts in standardization of image acquisition and analysis, psychoradiology is becoming a promising tool for the future of clinical care for patients with psychiatric disorders.

Resting state functional connectivity (RSFC) has been widely studied in functional magnetic resonance imaging (fMRI) and is observed by a significant temporal correlation of spontaneous low-frequency signal fluctuations (SLFs) both within and across hemispheres during rest. Different hypotheses of RSFC include the biophysical origin hypothesis and cognitive origin hypothesis, which show that the role of SLFs and RSFC is still not completely understood. Furthermore, RSFC and age studies have shown an "age-related compensation" phenomenon. RSFC data analysis methods include time domain analysis, seed-based correlation, regional homogeneity, and principal and independent component analyses. Despite advances in RSFC, the authors also discuss challenges and limitations, ranging from head motion to methodological limitations.

Psychiatric disorders are common and can be severe. There is a need to identify biomarkers of psychiatric disorders to better diagnose and treat patients with psychiatric symptoms. Magnetic resonance spectroscopy (MRS) is a tool used to measure the levels of various metabolites in the human brain, and MRS studies of psychiatric disorders have identified potentially useful biomarkers of psychiatric illness. There have been significant advances in the way that psychiatric disorders are understood, classified, and researched as well as improvements in magnetic resonance imaging/MRS technology. MRS as a tool has not yet proved helpful to individual patients with psychiatric symptoms.

> Despite considerable research evidence demonstrating significant neurobiological alterations in psychiatric disorders, incorporating neuroimaging approaches into clinical practice remains challenging. There is an urgent need for biologically validated psychiatric disease constructs that can inform diagnostic algorithms and targeted treatment development. In this article, the authors present a conceptual review of the most robust and impactful findings from studies that use neuroimaging methods in efforts to define distinct disease subtypes, while emphasizing cross-diagnostic and dimensional approaches. In addition, they discuss current challenges in psychoradiology and outline potential future strategies for clinically applicable translation.

> In neuroimaging research, averaging data at the level of the group results in blurring of potentially meaningful individual differences. A more widespread use of an individual-specific approach is advocated for, which involves a more thorough investigation of each individual in a group, and characterization of idiosyncrasies at the level of behavior, cognition, and symptoms, as well as at the level of brain organization. It is hoped that such an approach, focused on individuals, will provide convergent findings that will help identify the underlying pathologic condition in various psychiatric disorders and help in the development of treatments individualized for each patient.

> The application of personalized medicine to psychiatry is challenging. Psychoradiology could provide biomarkers based on objective tests in support of the diagnostic classifications and treatment planning. The authors review potential psychoradiological biomarkers for psychopharmaceutical effects. Although none of the biomarkers reviewed are yet of sufficient clinical utility to inform the selection of a specific pharmacologic compound for an individual patient, there is strong consensus that advanced multimodal approaches will contribute to discovery of novel treatment predictors in psychiatric disorders. Progress has been sufficient to warrant enthusiasm, in which application of neuroimaging-based biomarkers would represent a paradigm shift and modernization of psychiatric practice.

> MR imaging is a suitable instrument for the detection of incidental radiological findings in patients with early psychosis and guidance of subsequent treatment adjustments. The authors outline evidence showing the clinical utility of MR imaging to guide treatment selection by identifying radiological abnormalities and predicting clinical outcomes in early-stage psychosis. They argue that MR imaging is an indispensable screening tool to detect gross radiological abnormalities in early psychosis and implementation in routine clinical assessments is warranted. The authors highlight future key challenges and make pragmatic suggestions to exploit the potential of MR imaging to construct robust prognostic models for personalized early interventions.

Schizophrenia is a chronic psychotic disorder with a lifetime prevalence of about 1%. Onset is typically in adolescence or early adulthood; characteristic symptoms include positive symptoms, negative symptoms, and impairments in cognition. Neuroimaging studies have shown substantive evidence of brain structural, functional, and neurochemical alterations that are more pronounced in the association cortex and subcortical regions. These abnormalities are not sufficiently specific to be of diagnostic value, but there may be a role for imaging techniques to provide predictions of outcome. Incorporating multimodal imaging datasets using machine learning approaches may offer better diagnostic and predictive value in schizophrenia.

Major depression is common and debilitating. Identifying neurobiological subtypes that comprise the disorder and predict clinical outcome are key challenges. Genetic and environmental factors leading to major depression are expressed in neural structure and function. Volumetric decreases in gray matter have been demonstrated in corticolimbic circuits involved in emotion regulation. MR imaging observable abnormalities reflect cytoarchitectonic alterations within a local neuroendocrine milieu with systemic effects. Multivariate pattern analysis offers the potential to identify the neurobiological subtypes and predictors of clinical outcome. It is essential to characterize disease heterogeneity by incorporating data-driven inductive and symptom-based deductive approaches in an iterative process.

Autism spectrum disorder (ASD) emerges during early childhood and is marked by a relatively narrow window in which infants transition from exhibiting normative behavioral profiles to displaying the defining features of the ASD phenotype in toddlerhood. Prospective brain imaging studies in infants at high familial risk for autism have revealed important insights into the neurobiology and developmental unfolding of ASD. In this article, the authors review neuroimaging studies of brain development in ASD from birth through toddlerhood, relate these findings to candidate neurobiological mechanisms, and discuss implications for future research and translation to clinical practice.

This review summarizes current knowledge obtained from psychoradiological studies of posttraumatic stress disorder (PTSD). The authors first focus on 3 key anatomic structures (hippocampus, amygdala, and medial prefrontal cortex) and the functional circuits to which they contribute. In addition, they discuss the triple-network model, a widely accepted neurobiological model of PTSD that explains the vast majority of neuroimaging findings, as well as their interactions and relationships to functional disruptions in PTSD.

Foreword
Psychoradiology

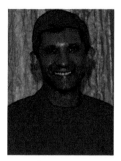

Suresh K. Mukherji, MD, MBA, FACR
Consulting Editor

So, one of the reasons I decided not to go into psychiatry was that I found the criteria for diagnosing various psychiatric disorders very ambiguous. The criteria for arriving at a specific diagnosis were based on the *Diagnostic and Statistical Manual of Mental Disorders* (*DSM*). It was *DSM-III* when I was medical school, and the current edition is *DSM-V*. I think every medical student felt that they had characteristics of every psychiatric disorder after they finished their psychiatry clerkship!

The development of MR imaging brought much promise to help provide objective criteria and better clarity to discriminate between different psychiatric diseases that had overlapping *DSM* criteria. Unfortunately, we were unable to make much progress by the images alone. However, the new era of advanced quantitative techniques, novel image acquisition strategies, and semiautomated quantitative image analysis approaches have identified promising imaging biomarkers to quantitatively identify various mental disorders. These early results form the basis of the US National Institute of Mental Health's Research Domain Criteria initiative to investigate psychiatric imaging for diagnosis heralded the field of "psychoradiology."

I wish to thank Dr Qiyong Gong, MD, PhD for agreeing to edit this issue on the clinical aims of "psychoradiology". As an internationally recognized leader in psychoradiology, Dr Gong has created a wonderful issue based on the contributions of international experts in this emerging field. I thank all the authors for their outstanding contributions. This translational issue will benefit all individuals who care for patients with these challenging and complex disorders.

One of the many "fun" decisions editors make is to determine if their upcoming issue will help "predict the future" or help "create the future" of their specialty. This issue of *Neuroimaging Clinics* on "psychoradiology" is a veiled attempt to help "create the future" by presenting a thought-provoking issue that highlights the possibilities of advanced MR technique to quantitatively and objectively diagnose a variety of psychiatric disorders. I thank Dr Gong for his willingness and tenacity to tackle such a bold and challenging topic.

Suresh K. Mukherji, MD, MBA, FACR
Clinical Professor
Marian University
Director of Head & Neck Radiology
ProScan Imaging
Regional Medical Director
Envision Physician Services
Carmel, Indiana, USA

E-mail address:
sureshmukherji@hotmail.com

neuroimaging.theclinics.com

Preface
Clinical Aims of Psychoradiology

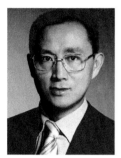

Qiyong Gong, MD, PhD
Editor

In the past 2 decades, radiological imaging techniques have rapidly evolved to become powerful tools in studying the human brain in both healthy and diseased conditions. For psychiatry, this is particularly true with the advances of MR imaging, where the development of the multi-modal MR imaging has allowed quantification of brain tissue at the structural, functional, and molecular levels. While early experience using brain scans in psychiatry with traditional visual image inspection failed to establish meaningful benefit to patient care, improved and novel image acquisition strategies and semi-automated quantitative image analysis approaches have established the clinical relevance of brain imaging studies of psychiatric patients. Using these advances, the field of Psychoradiology has developed to utilize neuroimaging approaches to advance differential diagnosis and individualized patient care for common psychiatric illnesses. Given the high prevalence of psychiatric disorders and the potential impact on work flow and training programs in Radiology of this evolving field, the aim of this series of articles will be to summarize these developments, describe future challenges, and spur involvement of radiologists in optimally advancing this fast-evolving field.

Using high-field MR imaging (ie, 3.0 Tesla MR), the structural and functional correlates of a number of psychiatric disorders have been identified. Taking advantage of new approaches and techniques for the acquisition and analysis of the imaging data, numerous clinical studies have revealed imaging biomarkers for mental disorders and clarified their pathologic mechanisms. Other studies have identified MR imaging biomarkers associated with risk for developing mental disorders prior to their emergence, which is important for illness prevention strategies. The results support the current focus on the biological investigation of mental disorders advocated by the US National Institute of Mental Health's Research Domain Criteria initiative and provide the basis for a major step toward the translational use of psychiatric imaging for diagnosis, prediction of treatment response, and monitoring therapeutic interventions.

In this issue, we invited internationally renowned experts in the emerging field of psychoradiology, including individuals who developed the imaging data acquisition and sophisticated analytical methods, to review and discuss the state of their fields as pertains to radiological applications for psychiatry. This issue will also contain selected clinical applications of psychoradiology for the major neuropsychiatric illnesses. In the first section of contributions, following an overview of the field of psychoradiology, the major psychiatric imaging methods will be reviewed, including resting state functional MRI imaging and MR spectroscopy. Then, state-of-the-art image analysis protocols for psychiatry are reviewed. This will cover structural and functional brain imaging analysis, and the connectome analysis for psychiatric illnesses. The second section will discusses the most general issues related to subtyping heterogeneous psychiatric syndromes, monitoring and predicting treatment

Neuroimag Clin N Am 30 (2020) xvii–xviii
https://doi.org/10.1016/j.nic.2019.09.013
1052-5149/20/© 2019 Published by Elsevier Inc.

neuroimaging.theclinics.com

response using imaging biomarkers. Finally, in the third section, the applications of psychiatric imaging to common psychiatric disorders, including schizophrenia, major depression, bipolar disorder, autism spectrum disorder, and attention deficit hyperactivity disorder, will be reviewed to provide an up-to-date review of clinically useful developments relevant to each of these disorders.

We hope the proposed issue brings greater awareness of the emerging and promising field of psychoradiology. In contrast to other traditional radiology subspecialties, psychoradiological techniques (ie, clinical psychiatric imaging) involve the use of both qualitative and quantitative "radiological signs" (ie, imaging biomarkers) of mental disorders. These could be utilized in a clinical context similar to the current methods that neuroradiologists use to manage neurologic diseases. In particular, the development of fast multimodal imaging facilities, standardization of imaging data acquisition and quality control, and the efficient and increasingly semi-

automated computational models for image analysis will expedite the translation of psychoradiological discoveries into patient care. And, hopefully it will inspire some of the best young minds in our field to contribute to progress in this field.

Qiyong Gong, MD, PhD
Clinical Professor of Radiology
Director of Huaxi MR Research Center (HMRRC)
Section of Neuroradiology
Department of Radiology
West China Hospital of Sichuan University
Chengdu, Sichuan Province, China

President
Shenjing Hospital of China Medical University
Shenyang, Liaoning Province, China

Associate Editor
American Journal of Psychiatry

E-mail address:
qiyonggong@hmrrc.org.cn

Clinical Strategies and Technical Challenges in Psychoradiology

Fei Li, MD, PhD[a,b,1], Dongsheng Wu, MD[a,b,1], Su Lui, MD, PhD[a,b,*],
Qiyong Gong, MD, PhD[a,b], John A. Sweeney, PhD[c]

KEYWORDS

- Psychoradiology • Psychiatric disorders • Magnetic resonance imaging • Imaging acquisition
- Imaging analysis • Clinical application • Neuroimaging

KEY POINTS

- The biological heterogeneity of psychiatric syndromes and neurobiological mechanisms underpinning radiological abnormalities need to be addressed and further investigated.
- Proper examination procedures, including optimal image acquisition, rigorous image quality control, standardized image processing, and individualized analysis, are essential for psychoradiology.
- Psychoradiology has the potential to play an important role in clinical diagnosis, evaluation of treatment response and prognosis, and illness risk prediction for patients with psychiatric disorders.
- Clinical challenges remain for improving psychoradiological utility and validity.

INTRODUCTION

Psychoradiology is an emerging discipline at the intersection between radiology and psychiatry. It applies radiological technologies to unveil patterns of anatomic and functional brain changes in patients with psychiatric disorders in vivo. It holds promise for playing a key role in clinical diagnosis, evaluation of treatment response, prediction of prognosis, and illness risk prediction for patients with psychiatric disorders.[1] Although psychoradiology was formally described by Lui and colleagues in 2016,[1] the idea of developing imaging biomarkers for psychiatric disorders dates back to 1976, when the first study revealed an enlarged ventricular size in patients with schizophrenia.[2]

Gong and colleagues and other investigators have since developed the psychoradiological hypothesis of mental disorders, theorizing that brain structural and functional connectivity alterations lead to clinical symptoms and syndromes.[1,3–5] Well-replicated radiological observations[6] have played a major role in the shift from seeing serious mental illnesses in psychological terms as problems of adaptation to life circumstances to the current view that they represent brain disorders.[7–9]

This effort has accelerated to a great degree within the past 20 years due to the rapid and extensive development of magnetic resonance imaging (MRI), molecular imaging, and other diagnostic imaging techniques. In particular, new MRI

Disclosure Statement: All the authors have no conflicts of interest to disclose.
[a] Huaxi MR Research Center (HMRRC), Department of Radiology, West China Hospital of Sichuan University, No. 37 Guo Xue Lane, Chengdu 610041, China; [b] Psychoradiology Research Unit of Chinese Academy of Medical Sciences, West China Hospital of Sichuan University, No. 37 Guo Xue Lane, Chengdu 610041, China; [c] Department of Psychiatry and Behavioral Neuroscience, University of Cincinnati, Suite 3200, 260 Stetson Street, Cincinnati, OH 45219, USA
[1] F. Li and D. Wu contributed equally to this work.
* Corresponding author. Huaxi MR Research Center (HMRRC), Department of Radiology, West China Hospital of Sichuan University, No. 37 Guo Xue Lane, Chengdu 610041, China.
E-mail address: lusuwcums@tom.com

Neuroimag Clin N Am 30 (2020) 1–13
https://doi.org/10.1016/j.nic.2019.09.001

technologies, such as high-resolution structural MRI, perfusion mapping, magnetic resonance spectroscopy (MRS), diffusion tensor imaging (DTI), and blood oxygenation level–dependent (BOLD) functional MRI (fMRI), have given rise to an increasing body of scientific literature that elucidates how various psychiatric syndromes are associated with alterations in brain structures and function across time and with treatment.

Multiple imaging biomarkers have been identified in different psychiatric disorders, among which some have shown potential clinical utility for subtyping, prediction, and evaluation. Although the clinical use of psychoradiology is already in sight, there are still issues and challenges that need to be addressed before wide-scale clinical application. In particular, the clinical strategies for examining patients, analyzing images, and using findings to help clinical work need to be better validated and optimized.

STRATEGY FOR EXAMINATIONS

Like other imaging examinations, the first step of psychoradiology is to choose proper techniques for managing patients. Unlike tumor, stroke, and most neurologic diseases, brain abnormalities in psychiatric disorders are subtle and often involve functional alterations that contribute to cognitive and emotional disturbances. As a result, psychoradiology approaches require multimodal imaging techniques, especially high spatial resolution structural MRI, DTI, fMRI, perfusion-weighted imaging, MRS, electroencephalography, and positron emission tomography (PET). Multimodal imaging techniques requires clinical balance between the number of the techniques needed for particular patients or disorders and their cost. As in neurologic disorders, high-resolution T1-weighted imaging (T1WI) is used for detecting anatomic gray matter abnormality, DTI for white matter deficits, resting-state fMRI (rs-fMRI) for brain dysfunction identification, and MRS for neurometabolic information.

A second question pertains to which patients need psychoradiological examination. Given the current state of knowledge, anyone with a suspected serious mental illness may benefit from an imaging examination, not only for ruling out other diseases, such as inflammation or tumor, but also as a baseline for subtyping and following treatment response. The clinical high-risk population, individuals with strong familial liability or prodromal manifestations of illness, also may benefit from an imaging examination to objectively assess risk and guide initiation of preventive interventions. Another issue is whether sedation or even anesthesia is needed for evaluating patients. A large majority of patients can cooperate with examination, sometimes with the help of mental health staff and relatives. In cases of some children or acutely ill manic patients, however, sedation may be needed, although sedating medications can affect imaging features, especially fMRI.[10] The safety of the patient needs to be an important consideration as in other imaging examinations. To reduce patient distress and increase cooperation, it can be advantageous to have a psychiatrist, psychologist, or relative accompany patients to scan sessions and, if needed, be with patients during an examination. A quiet ready room is helpful for preparing patients for examination and a mock scanner may be helpful to prepare patients. Magnetic resonance (MR)-compatible monitoring devices, such as an eye tracking system, are useful not only for monitoring patient safety but also for monitoring head position and collecting data about eye movements that have an impact on fMRI data.[11–13] Usually, the time for 1 MR examination is best limited to 40 minutes to 60 to maintain patient comfort and safety and optimize acquired image quality.

Image quality control in psychoradiology is stricter than in other radiology disciplines because both structural and functional quantitative analyses are needed. In addition to general quality control, the control of the signal-to-noise ratio (SNR),[14] the contrast-to-noise ratio (CNR), and image uniformity are required.[15] For example, when acquiring T1WI, the image interpolation function should be turned off, the acceleration factor should not exceed 2, and T2-weighted images with the same resolution should be acquired for better accuracy of brain surface reconstruction.[16] For DTI, the acceleration factors of 2 to 3 might be optimal, and the use of cardiac gating would be helpful in minimizing the tissue pulsation secondary to the cardiac cycle.[17] In rs-fMRI acquisition, an electrocardiogram needs to be acquired simultaneously for the correction of cardiac cycle effects on BOLD signals. The incorporation of a gradient-echo acquisition also can be useful in generating phase and magnitude images simultaneously that can be used for correcting or visualizing distortions caused by susceptibility and inhomogeneous fields.[18,19] The acquisition of MRS data requires precise anatomic location of regions of interest (ROIs). For psychoradiology, the main focus shifts from visual inspection of images to quantitative analysis, leading to many of these requirements for image acquisition.

STRATEGY FOR IMAGE ANALYSIS

Unlike traditional qualitative diagnostic proced-ures in clinical radiology, psychoradiology is performed in a quantitative way. Thus, postpro-cessing is necessary after image acquisition. Although tools for such analysis are rapidly evolving, there is no guideline for the integrated analysis of multimodel imaging, which remains a challenge for the clinical application of psychor-adiology. In this issue, some detailed strategies for data analysis are presented in the following chapters.

In brief, for T1WI, there are 2 common methods for structural MRI postprocessing, voxel-based analysis (VBA) and surface-based morphologic (SBM) analysis. Voxel-based morphometry (VBM) analysis can be conducted via Statistical Para-metric Mapping (SPM) (http://www.fil.ion.ucl.ac.uk/spm/), and the most commonly used method is diffeomorphic anatomical registration through exponentiated Lie algebra (DARTEL).[20–22] Basic procedures include segmentation of gray/white matter and cerebrospinal fluid, creation of DARTEL templates (6 templates through an 18 iteration process), registration of all individual deformations to the DARTEL template (the sixth template is the clearest for standard Montreal Neurological Institute space), and smoothing (usu-ally with a full-width at half-maximum [FWHM] gaussian kernel of 8 mm to 12 mm).[23] The smoothed image allows for intergroup compari-sons of gray matter density and gray matter vol-ume; the image after modulation represents gray matter volume, and the unmodulated image repre-sents gray matter density. In subsequent statistical analyses, the whole-brain volume of each subject is acquired as a covariate for comparison between groups to eliminate the effects of individual differ-ences in total brain volume, and for comparison of individual patient values with normative data. SBM analysis is usually performed using FreeSur-fer (http://surfer.nmr.mgh.harvard.edu) or CIVET (developed by the McConnell Brain Imaging Centre). The standard procedures of image pre-processing with FreeSurfer include head motion correction, removal of nonbrain tissue,[24–26] auto-mated transformation to standard Talairach space, segmentation of the subcortical white mat-ter and deep gray matter volumetric structures, in-tensity normalization,[27] tessellation of gray matter and white matter boundary, automated topology correction,[26,28] and surface deformation following intensity gradients to optimally place the gray/white matter and gray matter/cerebrospinal fluid borders where the greatest shift in intensity de-fines the transition to the other tissue class.[29]

FreeSurfer automatically applies different FWHM (ie, 10 mm, 15 mm, 20 mm, or 25 mm) gaussian smoothing kernels for later statistical analysis. In statistical analysis, between-group comparisons have been performed with the general linear model method, which can include features, such as sex and age, as covariates.[30] Cortical thickness, sur-face area, sulcal features (the number, depth, and frequency) and brain asymmetry can also be quantified.

In DTI, by using tract-based spatial statistics (TBSS) and VBA, parameters, including fractional anisotropy (FA), mean diffusivity, packing density, myelination, and axon diameter, can be quantified to assess changes of the physical properties of white matter bundles. VBA registers all data of the subject (including gray matter and cerebrospi-nal fluid) into a standard space and performs sta-tistical analyses on each voxel of the brain; then, it locates brain regions with altered parameters. The image data preprocessing and statistical anal-ysis of VBA can be achieved by SPM version 2 and above. TBSS examines the whole brain without prespecifying tracts of interest for estimating localized change in FA by constructing average FA fiber skeleton maps of all subjects first and then registering all FA images of from patients on it to identify altered white matter tracts. TBSS combines the strengths of both VBAs with those of tractography-based analyses, thus avoiding the problem of inaccurate positioning caused by inaccurate image registration and smoothing. It can quantitatively and objectively evaluate white matter structure. Additionally, by using tractogra-phy, graph theory analyses can be performed to comprehensively evaluate white matter connectiv-ity in the brain.[31–33]

Rs-fMRI focuses on spontaneous changes in the BOLD signal in a resting state or task-negative state. In addition to regular data prepro-cessing, slice time correction, motion correction, spatial normalization, and spatial smoothing are required. The time series needs to be bandpass filtered to assess a particular frequency band of in-terest (eg, 0.01–0.08 Hz) to eliminate influences of low-frequency signal drift and high-frequency noise caused by respiration and heartbeat and to extract low-frequency signal oscillations that reflect spontaneous activity of the brain.[34] Post-processing typically is carried out in 1 of 2 ways: (1) the synchronization analysis of low-frequency oscillations between different brain regions for functional connectivity analyses,[35] which is used to identify connectivity alterations in neural net-works, such as in the default mode network,[33,36] and (2) the regional characteristic analysis of the low-frequency oscillations. The amplitude of low-frequency fluctuation, fractional amplitude of low-frequency fluctuation, and regional homogeneity are commonly used as indicators to investigate the characteristics of low frequency oscillations in local brain regions.

MRS noninvasively detects and quantifies neurometabolites, such as N-acetylaspartate (NAA) (a putative marker of neuronal viability), choline (Cho) (a marker for membrane integrity and phospholipid metabolism), creatine (Cr) (a marker for energy metabolism), myoinositol (ml) (an astroglial marker), γ-aminobutyric acid (an inhibitory neurotransmitter in mammalian brain), and glutamate or/and glutamine (related to excitatory neurotransmission). One common finding in depression is the reduction of NAA in temporal and hippocampal regions. Other findings included reductions in NAA/Cr, NAA/Cho, and NAA/(Cr plus Cho). For example, the NAA/Cr ratio in prefrontal cortex of individuals with depression has been shown to be significantly lower than that of healthy individuals, with this deficit being greater in moderate than mild depression. Detailed information is provided in John D. Port's article, "Magnetic Resonance Spectroscopy for Psychiatry: Progress in the Last Decade," in this issue. These quantitative results may be useful for clinical work.

STRATEGY FOR CLINICAL APPLICATION

Although traditional MRI is widely used to detect tumors or inflammation in patients with psychiatric disorders, the subtle brain abnormalities associated with psychiatric disorders have been noninvasively identified with advanced radiological technologies. Numerous basic, preclinical, and clinical studies have revealed a series of imaging biomarkers of brain structural and functional abnormalities. These studies have greatly promoted understanding of the pathologic mechanisms of abnormal brain structure and function in psychiatric disorders. The clinical value of imaging biomarkers for the most common psychiatric disorders, such as major depressive disorder, schizophrenia, posttraumatic stress disorder, and autism spectrum disorder, are presented in the later chapters of Section Three. In this article, strategies for clinical use are summarized. Generally, psychoradiological biomarkers considered in isolation have not yet been validated for making patient care decisions for individual patients; however, they can visually show psychiatrists and patients subtle structural and functional changes and in the near future help assist doctors in differential diagnosis, treatment planning, and prediction of illness course.

Diagnosis and Subtyping

Psychiatric disorders traditionally have been diagnosed and classified on the basis of broad syndromes defined by patients' and parents' reports and behavioral observations rather than on the basis of their underlying neurobiological substrates. As a result, psychiatric syndromes are heterogeneous and they biologically overlap,[37] limiting the success of developing imaging and other biological biomarkers. Because this situation limits feasibility of identifying imaging biomarkers for different psychiatric syndromes, the field has moved in different directions, primarily toward developing objective psychoradiological biomarkers, such as structural features (alterations in gray matter/white matter volume, cortical morphometric features including thickness and surface area, and diffusion properties of white matter tracts) and functional features (activity and connectivity), which can facilitate early diagnosis and subtype patients into more biologically homogeneous groups. The US National Institute of Mental Health proposed the Research Domain Criteria project, with the aim to in part develop psychoradiological biomarkers for psychiatric disorders based on different dimensions of observable behaviors and neurobiological measures that are correlated to specific cognitive constructs across different brain systems.

For example, Sun and colleagues[38] made 1 of the first efforts to subtype psychiatric disorders based on imaging features, and 2 distinct schizophrenia subtypes were identified using DTI. Using fMRI in a multisite sample, it was shown that patients with major depressive disorder can be divided into 4 neurophysiological subtypes (biotypes) by distinct patterns of dysfunctional connectivity in limbic and frontostriatal networks. Clustering patients on this basis led to high sensitivity and specificity (82%–93%) in the development of diagnostic classifiers for depression subtypes with multisite validation and out-of-sample replication data sets.[39] Similar studies have revealed new biotypes in schizophrenia, attention-deficit/hyperactivity disorder (ADHD), bipolar disorder, and other psychiatric disorders,[37,40–42] which highlights the potential application for psychoradiology to help subtype patients with psychiatric disorders based on objective imaging markers rather than observation of behavior and symptom profiles and for using these classifications to better individualize patient care in parallel with development of optimal treatment strategies for the identified subgroups.

Guiding Therapeutic Intervention and Interventional Psychoradiology

Psychoradiological biomarkers can be of importance in guiding treatment of patients with psychiatric disorders by helping clinicians make difficult differential diagnoses and select optimal treatment procedures and targets for subgroups of patients with particular neurobiological abnormalities. Psychoradiological biomarkers also may help predict psychiatric disorders in at-risk individuals so that primary prevention approaches can be implemented for those who most need them, so patients likely to be refractory to first-line treatments can be identified before beginning treatment, and so that the fundamental understanding of causal neural mechanisms of illness can be identified to spur development of novel treatments.[43–47]

For example, studies have identified a distributed pattern of brain activity reflected in fMRI responses during fear conditioning, which can discriminate patients with panic disorder who responded to cognitive behavioral therapy from those who did not with 82% accuracy.[45] Using resting-state functional connectivity analyses, other studies discovered that disrupted functional connectivity mainly in thalamocortical circuits is correlated to refractory depression, whereas more widespread decreased functional connectivity in the limbic-striatal-pallidal-thalamic circuit is associated with nonrefractory depression.[43] Imaging biomarkers also could provide valuable information about treatment targets.[3,48] For example, regions including prefrontal cortex and striatum receive robust dopaminergic projections, which are believed to be implicated in the pathogenesis of schizophrenia. Hypofunction of the medial prefrontal cortex as well as hyperactivity of the hippocampus and striatum, in patients with schizophrenia may in time provide psychoradiological biomarkers for the targets of treatment.[3]

These findings demonstrate promising new evidence that psychoradiological biomarkers may provide valuable information in monitoring and predicting treatment response, which could be of great importance in detecting patients at an early stage who require adjunctive medical and psychosocial therapies, because they may not respond to first-line treatments, and those likely to recover without any intervention, by optimizing timing, intensity, and form of therapeutic intervention.

Prediction of Illness Onset

Predicting the onset of illness for a high-risk person is another important role of psychoradiology. Psychoradiological studies have suggested that the brain's structure and function are different between high-risk individuals who subsequently develop psychosis and individuals who do not.[49–52] For example, using multiparadigm fMRI data to investigate network-level changes in functional connectome of the human brain, Cao and colleagues[51] found an individual-specific "trait" abnormality in brain architecture characterized as increased connectivity in the cerebello-thalamo-cortical circuitry in individuals at clinical high risk for psychosis. This is a pattern that is significantly more pronounced among those who develop psychosis than those who do not among high-risk individuals. This abnormality is significantly associated with thought disorder and predictive of time to conversion.

These findings highlight the potential for psychoradiology to help identify those at high risk for developing psychosis to predict who will later convert to a disease state in advance of its onset. This knowledge can indicate a need for those at greatest risk for early preventive pharmacologic and psychological interventions, while sparing those with lower conversion risk of unnecessary exposure to treatment side effects. These advances could help optimize allocation of clinical resources in mental health care systems.

The workflow pipeline of psychoradiology in clinical practice is summarized in **Fig. 1**.

FUTURE CHALLENGES

Although psychoradiology has great promise as a clinical discipline aiding in the diagnosis and treatment of psychiatric patients, there are still many issues and challenges in this growing field that need to be addressed before routine clinical application.

Problems in Clinical Translation

First, MRI-based brain volume measurements can be influenced by various technical parameters, especially when reliability and reproducibility are critical for clinical translation in psychoradiology. For instance, the number of head coil channels,[53] inconsistent subject positioning,[54] inconsistent image contrast,[55] and differences in MR scanner vendors, and field strength[56] can have an impact on on interpretation of quantitative image characteristics. Heterogeneity of MRI scanning parameters across studies and sites in voxel size, number of diffusion directions, and slice thickness may have resulted in decreased reliability of functional and structural MRI studies in psychiatric disorders.[56–58] These differences are difficult to eliminate by statistical means. Homogenization of technical considerations becomes more crucial with the introduction of multiple MRI scanners, in a

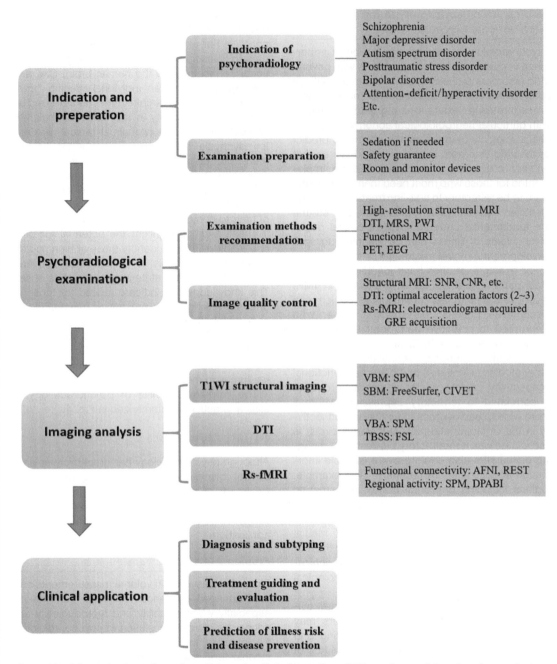

Fig. 1. Workflow pipeline of psychoradiology in clinical practice. AFNI, analyses of functional neuroimages; DPABI, data processing and analysis for brain imaging; EEG, electroencephalography; FSL, FMRIB software library; GRE, gradient echo; PWI, perfusion-weighted imaging; REST, resting-state fMRI data analysis toolkit.

situation where multicenter trials or cross-site application of a diagnostic or predictive algorithm are used. Kruggel and colleagues[59] compared different scanner platforms of 1.5T and 3.0T and found that different levels of image quality, regarding SNR, CNR, and combined information of the joint histogram limited the consistency of brain volume measurements. Hence, data from different scanning protocols and platforms must be carefully considered to avoid confounding the true effects of interest with variability among scanning platforms. Also, this issue highlights the need to establish optimal acquisition parameters for specific clinical applications.

An early study[60] in schizophrenia with fMRI suggested that factors of variation (both artifactual and intrinsic) could be controlled to improve test-retest reliability. Zhao and colleagues[61] analyzed data from 21 subjects who underwent 2 scans within 2 weeks on a 3T MRI scanner from General Electric (Milwaukee, United States) and the third visit on a 3T MRI scanner from Siemens approximately 8 months later for assessment of intrascanner and interscanner reliability of rs-fMRI based on voxelwise whole-brain analytical metrics. The rs-fMRI results[61,62] indicated that the data were reliable within the same scanner, whereas inter-canner reliability was a more significant factor when data were compared across platforms and field strength. Data, including MRI-derived measurements in a longitudinal morphometric study of human brains,[61,63] were trustworthy at a single 1.5T site, even with different sequences or after upgrading systems; nevertheless, the reliability should be carefully considered when images are collected across vendors and/or field strength.[62] Changes in scanner hardware can lead to the introduction of different bias effects in the brain analyses, whereas intervendor changes generally exerted greater effects compared with intravendor scanner changes.[59] In the context of quantitative analysis to detect relatively subtle brain alterations, consideration of the impact of technical factors in multisite research and in developing widely useful normative data are particularly important.

The acquisition of structural MRI and fMRI data is costly, especially regarding the time involved in postprocessing. Furthermore, the quality of MRI data is affected by many factors, including head motion, and physiologic factors, such as heart beating and breathing, are critical biological confounds. This is especially with fMRI, where cardiopulmonary function, age and sex effects, and anatomic variability have an impact on data interpretation.[63,64] Thus, individual patient variability and protocol/scanner factors are critical for clinical application.

Therefore, it is imperative to establish standardized data acquisition and image quality control solutions. To address heterogeneity between different centers/sequences, a standardized MRI sequence is needed that can generate images with similar properties concerning SNR, CNR, voxel size, and slice thickness, regardless of the scanner platform and manufacturer. Homogeneous data acquisition and analysis can be provided by a specific protocol across sites, like that developed by the Alzheimer's Disease Neuroimaging Initiative consortium.[65] Even with these efforts, heterogeneities based on site still exist for

complicated reasons.[66] Multitask learning has been deployed to simultaneously learn the features of site-shared and site-specific features extracted from multicenter MRI data of brain morphology. Neuroimaging studies have demonstrated the advantages of multitask learning to decode brain alterations and for classifying disease.[67,68]

Second, it is necessary to develop stable and efficient semiautomated computational approaches for image analysis. Studies of brain morphometry[69,70] initially used morphometric measurements obtained from brain regions with manual delineation of ROIs. This ROI-based method sometimes encountered difficulties under certain conditions for the delineation of unambiguous structures, such as the hippocampi or the ventricles. VBAs and surface-based analyses can be used to identify whole-brain changes[71]; these analyses are automated, relatively easy-to-use, time-efficient tools and have been widely used in psychiatric research.[72–74] Such approaches can also shorten the duration of the evaluation pipeline to speed availability of feedback to referring physicians. The recent development of psychoradiological tools to detect the individual-specific biomarkers in patients with psychotic disorders has been extremely exciting.[75,76] Although reliable, fully automated, standardized methods can improve implementation across different sites with a unified software platform, an individualized approach can be implemented as suited for specific purposes.[77] Standardized pipelines for preprocessing MRI data are becoming increasingly sophisticated, such as improved sequences linked to the Human Connectome Project.[78]

Third, the development of fast multimodal imaging facilities is important. To discover robust neuroimaging biomarkers for diagnosis and patient stratification, multicenter and multimodal studies are becoming popular, thereby increasing sample size and providing detailed imaging features of psychosis patients.[79] Multimodal imaging, which can combine structural MRI, DTI, fMRI, and even PET data together, can scan subjects with a variety of sequences to acquire structural, functional, and metabolic data of the brain in a single session.[80,81] It is a challenge for psychoradiologists to interpret these combined data sets acquired from variable combinations of different imaging modalities and methodologies, but machine learning approaches offer promise for usefully organizing multimodal data.

A method was specifically developed to analyze multimodal imaging data by Radua and colleagues.[82] This technique is a voxel-wise multimodal meta-analysis applied to anatomic and fMRI examinations in first-episode psychosis patients. This meta-analysis identified both structural and functional abnormalities in the brain as well as heterogeneity between studies. To speed up the reconstruction of images, Xiang and colleagues[83] fused multimodal MR acquisitions through deep learning. This deep learning approach reconstructed a 3-dimensional T2WI volume from the T1WI data and undersampled T2WI images. This approach was applied to data sets acquired by different MR vendors, and it showed excellent transferring capability. These approaches open the way for faster and more efficient multimodal image acquisition in clinical settings.

Pathophysiology of Imaging Signs

In addition to the challenges of particular imaging techniques, the unclear pathophysiology of imaging biomarkers is another challenge when explaining the meaning of brain imaging findings. Until this is resolved, psychoradiology will remain an empirical or actuarial field.

For example, in vivo neuroimaging studies[84,85] have supported the hypotheses that cortical glutamate dysfunction has an impact on subcortical dopamine synthesis capacity, which is a leading theory of the pathogenesis of schizophrenia. It is unclear, however, how alterations in in vivo cortical glutamate and dopamine levels and function result in the pathophysiology of psychosis. PET studies have shown that multiple neurochemical systems and molecular mechanisms can play roles in the pathophysiology of psychosis in the early course of the syndrome.[86,87] In terms of correlations between brain activation and behavior using task-based fMRI (studying brain activity as a particular cognitive, motor or emotion task is performed) to study individual differences, it is crucial that behavioral paradigms be optimized for clinical application. These studies can be effective in challenging brain circuitry of clinical interest and relating brain alterations to clinical features of interest, but add an additional layer of methods validation.

Region-specific structural changes in the rat cortex[88,89] after chronic antipsychotic treatment raise the issue that psychopharmacological treatments themselves can alter brain anatomy and function and thus have an impact on the use of algorithms for diagnosis and prediction. Postmortem structural studies in schizophrenia[90] found volume and cell number reduction in the pulvinar with stereological studies of the thalamus. This finding is in accordance with the view that thalamocortical dysfunction might play a role in schizophrenia because of the function of the thalamus as a key node in whole-brain neuronal circuits. This type of finding highlights the importance of network-level analysis of brain systems in studies of psychiatric illness. Structural imaging studies[91,92] provide evidence of volume reductions in bilateral thalami in schizophrenia that support the thalamocortical dysfunction hypothesis in patients with schizophrenia. Although understanding of the pathogenesis of psychosis remains limited, these initial results highlight the potential value of psychoradiology in better understanding the pathogenesis of serious mental illness and the translation of these findings into clinical practice.

Heterogeneity of Psychiatric Disorders

Psychiatric disorders are now diagnostically classified as broad syndromes defined based on patient complaints and behavioral observations.[1] The overlap of these syndromes in terms of illness presentation, genetics, neurobiology, and treatment response profiles remains large. This highlights the importance of psychoradiology not only for patient care but also as an important field working toward nosologic reorganization for diagnosis of serious mental illnesses based on biological features. In this latter effort, in vivo brain imaging can play a crucial role, to the great advantage of efforts to identify biologically discrete patient subgroups requiring specific therapies based on the nature of their brain disturbances.

Individuals with symptoms indicating that they are at risk for serious mental illness based on psychological assessment may share a phenotypic expression but one that results from different underlying brain abnormalities as suggested by recent large-scale multisite collaborative studies. For instance, autism spectrum disorder and schizophrenia share clinical features, including social withdrawal, theory of mind deficits, and sensory abnormalities.[93–95] It is not uncommon that several mental disorders show similar anatomic and functional deficits in brain networks including schizophrenia and bipolar disorder.[96] Psychiatric disorders share similar neurocognitive deficits[97] and overlapping features of emotional disorders.[1] Wang and colleagues[98] analyzed the multisite data set of patients with ADHD (ie, data from the ADHD-200[99]) with rs-fMRI based on 3 whole-brain VBA methods. Abnormal activity was found in some brain regions with the pooled data set; however, these results were highly heterogeneous across cohorts and within the same research center. The results from the study of multisite functional connectivity classification of autism[100] also indicated a poorer degree of accuracy of whole-brain functional connectivity in favor of heterogeneous features of connectivity disturbances with a particular spatial distribution in specific brain regions.

The clinical and imaging heterogeneity of psychiatric syndromes resulted in compromised specificity when assigning psychiatric disorders using machine learning approaches with MRI data. This has led many in psychiatric research to step back and conclude that the next step forward needs to be collecting large samples in multisite projects with dense phenotyping (including but not restricted to MRI) to identify biologically discrete patient groups, which can then be studied separately or stratified in clinical trials and genetic research. In this way, the clinical relevance of novel patient subgrouping approaches developed using MRI data can be evaluated. This is especially important as decades of patient subgrouping efforts based on psychological and behavioral features has produced limited gains. Until this issue of within diagnosis heterogeneity is resolved, the ability to identify MR biomarkers for diagnosis or guiding treatment decisions remains limited. The best way for psychoradiology to address this issue is to use psychoradiology and machine learning with prolonged imaging times, standardized acquisition strategies, advanced classification methodology, and large sample sizes to identify distinct patterns of brain abnormalities that run across and are not specific to particular psychiatric syndromes, and to define patterns of brain alterations and their relation to cognitive, affective, and behavioral clinical manifestations.[1]

This effort will require considerable interdisciplinary collaboration, from radiologists and physicists optimizing acquisition protocols, to statisticians and programmers developing rapid and automated measurement of brain features of interest, and to adiologists, psychiatrists, and psychologists working to translate new approaches into clinically useful contributions for improving psychiatric patient care.

SUMMARY

Psychoradiology is a young and evolving field. Research to date is already showing the utility of MRI data in psychiatry for facilitating clinical diagnosis, evaluation of treatment response and prognosis, identifying patient subgroups, and illness risk prediction. Further advances to translate these observations into clinical practice will require proper examination and validation of image acquisition and processing methods, rigorous image quality control, and standardized semiautomated image analysis. Addressing complex issues, such as the biological heterogeneity of psychiatric syndromes and unclear neurobiological mechanisms underpinning radiological abnormalities, is a challenge that needs to be resolved but one for which psychoradiology can make important contributions. With the advance of multimodal imaging and more efforts in standardization of image acquisition and analysis, psychoradiology has become a promising tool for the future of the clinical care of patients with psychiatric disorders.

ACKNOWLEDGMENTS

This study was supported by the National Natural Science Foundation of China (Grant Nos. 81671664, 81621003, 81761128023 and 81820108018). The authors acknowledge the support from Chang Jiang Scholars of China (Award Nos. T2014190, IRT16R52 and Q2015154), National Program for Support of Top-notch Young Professionals (National Program for Special Support of Eminent Professionals, Award No. W02070140) and the Functional and Molecular Imaging Key Laboratory of Sichuan Province (FMIKLSP, Grant: 2019JDS0044).

REFERENCES

1. Lui S, Zhou XJ, Sweeney JA, et al. Psychoradiology: the frontier of neuroimaging in psychiatry. Radiology 2016;281:357–72.
2. Johnstone EC, Crow TJ, Frith CD, et al. Cerebral ventricular size and cognitive impairment in chronic schizophrenia. Lancet 1976;2:924–6.
3. Gong Q, Lui S, Sweeney JA. A selective review of cerebral abnormalities in patients with first-episode schizophrenia before and after treatment. Am J Psychiatry 2016;173:232–43.
4. Tregellas J. Connecting brain structure and function in schizophrenia. Am J Psychiatry 2009;166:134–6.
5. Lui S, Deng W, Huang X, et al. Association of cerebral deficits with clinical symptoms in antipsychotic-naive first-episode schizophrenia: an optimized voxel-based morphometry and resting state functional connectivity study. Am J Psychiatry 2009; 166(2):196–205.
6. Klausner JD, Sweeney JA, Deck MD, et al. Clinical correlates of cerebral ventricular enlargement in schizophrenia. Further evidence for frontal lobe disease. J Nerv Ment Dis 1992;180:407–12.
7. Sarpal DK, Lencz T, Malhotra AK. In support of neuroimaging biomarkers of treatment response in first-episode schizophrenia. Am J Psychiatry 2016;173:732–3.

8. Port JD. Diagnosis of attention deficit hyperactivity disorder by using MR imaging and radiomics: a potential tool for clinicians. Radiology 2018;287: 631–2.

9. Gong Q. Response to Sarpal et al.: importance of neuroimaging biomarkers for treatment development and clinical practice. Am J Psychiatry 2016; 173:733–4.

10. Starbuck VN, Kay GG, Platenberg RC, et al. Functional magnetic resonance imaging reflects changes in brain functioning with sedation. Hum Psychopharmacol 2000;15:613–8.

11. Sweeney JA, Levy D, Harris MS. Commentary: eye movement research with clinical populations. Prog Brain Res 2002;140:507–22.

12. Rosano C, Krisky CM, Welling JS, et al. Pursuit and saccadic eye movement subregions in human frontal eye field: a high-resolution fMRI investigation. Cereb Cortex 2002;12:107–15.

13. Sweeney JA, Luna B, Keedy SK, et al. fMRI studies of eye movement control: investigating the interaction of cognitive and sensorimotor brain systems. Neuroimage 2007;36(Suppl 2): T54–60.

14. Yu S, Dai G, Wang Z, et al. A consistency evaluation of signal-to-noise ratio in the quality assessment of human brain magnetic resonance images. BMC Med Imaging 2018;18:17.

15. Jara JL, Saeed NP, Panerai RB, et al. Increasing the contrast-to-noise ratio of MRI signals for regional assessment of dynamic cerebral autoregulation. Acta Neurochir Suppl 2018;126: 153–7.

16. Misaki M, Savitz J, Zotev V, et al. Contrast enhancement by combining T1- and T2-weighted structural brain MR Images. Magn Reson Med 2015;74: 1609–20.

17. Yang E, Nucifora PG, Melhem ER. Diffusion MR imaging: basic principles. Neuroimaging Clin N Am 2011;21:1–25, vii.

18. Conklin CJ, Faro SH, Mohamed FB. Technical considerations for functional magnetic resonance imaging analysis. Neuroimaging Clin N Am 2014;24: 695–704.

19. Zaca D, Agarwal S, Gujar SK, et al. Special considerations/technical limitations of blood-oxygen-level-dependent functional magnetic resonance imaging. Neuroimaging Clin N Am 2014;24: 705–15.

20. Good CD, Johnsrude IS, Ashburner J, et al. A voxel-based morphometric study of ageing in 465 normal adult human brains. Neuroimage 2001;14:21–36.

21. Wright IC, McGuire PK, Poline JB, et al. A voxel-based method for the statistical analysis of gray and white matter density applied to schizophrenia. Neuroimage 1995;2:244–52.

22. Ashburner J. A fast diffeomorphic image registration algorithm. Neuroimage 2007;38:95–113.

23. Radua J, Canales-Rodriguez EJ, Pomarol-Clotet E, et al. Validity of modulation and optimal settings for advanced voxel-based morphometry. Neuroimage 2014;86:81–90.

24. Segonne F, Dale AM, Busa E, et al. A hybrid approach to the skull stripping problem in MRI. Neuroimage 2004;22:1060–75.

25. Fischl B, Salat DH, Busa E, et al. Whole brain segmentation: automated labeling of neuroanatomical structures in the human brain. Neuron 2002;33: 341–55.

26. Fischl B, van der Kouwe A, Destrieux C, et al. Automatically parcellating the human cerebral cortex. Cereb Cortex 2004;14:11–22.

27. Fischl B, Dale AM. Measuring the thickness of the human cerebral cortex from magnetic resonance images. Proc Natl Acad Sci U S A 2000;97: 11050–5.

28. Segonne F, Pacheco J, Fischl B. Geometrically accurate topology-correction of cortical surfaces using nonseparating loops. IEEE Trans Med Imaging 2007;26:518–29.

29. Jovicich J, Czanner S, Greve D, et al. Reliability in multi-site structural MRI studies: effects of gradient non-linearity correction on phantom and human data. Neuroimage 2006;30:436–43.

30. Fischl B, Sereno MI, Tootell RB, et al. High-resolution intersubject averaging and a coordinate system for the cortical surface. Hum Brain Mapp 1999;8:272–84.

31. Owen JP, Ziv E, Bukshpun P, et al. Test-retest reliability of computational network measurements derived from the structural connectome of the human brain. Brain Connect 2013;3:160–76.

32. van den Heuvel MP, Sporns O. Rich-club organization of the human connectome. J Neurosci 2011; 31:15775–86.

33. Hu ML, Zong XF, Mann JJ, et al. A review of the functional and anatomical default mode network in Schizophrenia. Neurosci Bull 2017;33:73–84.

34. Barry RL, Williams JM, Klassen LM, et al. Evaluation of preprocessing steps to compensate for magnetic field distortions due to body movements in BOLD fMRI. Magn Reson Imaging 2010;28: 235–44.

35. Bullmore E, Sporns O. Complex brain networks: graph theoretical analysis of structural and functional systems. Nat Rev Neurosci 2009;10:186–98.

36. Whitfield-Gabrieli S, Ford JM. Default mode network activity and connectivity in psychopathology. Annu Rev Clin Psychol 2012;8:49–76.

37. Clementz BA, Sweeney JA, Hamm JP, et al. Identification of distinct psychosis biotypes using brain-based biomarkers. Am J Psychiatry 2016;173: 373–84.

38. Sun H, Lui S, Yao L, et al. Two patterns of white matter abnormalities in medication-naive patients with first-episode schizophrenia revealed by diffusion tensor imaging and cluster analysis. JAMA Psychiatry 2015;72:678–86.

39. Drysdale AT, Grosenick L, Downar J, et al. Resting-state connectivity biomarkers define neurophysiological subtypes of depression. Nat Med 2017;23:28–38.

40. Insel TR, Cuthbert BN. Medicine. Brain disorders? Precisely. Science 2015;348:499–500.

41. Karalunas SL, Fair D, Musser ED, et al. Subtyping attention-deficit/hyperactivity disorder using temperament dimensions: toward biologically based nosologic criteria. JAMA Psychiatry 2014;71:1015–24.

42. Tamminga CA, Pearlson G, Keshavan M, et al. Bipolar and schizophrenia network for intermediate phenotypes: outcomes across the psychosis continuum. Schizophr Bull 2014;40(Suppl 2):S131–7.

43. Doehrmann O, Ghosh SS, Polli FE, et al. Predicting treatment response in social anxiety disorder from functional magnetic resonance imaging. JAMA Psychiatry 2013;70:87–97.

44. Hahn T, Kircher T, Straube B, et al. Predicting treatment response to cognitive behavioral therapy in panic disorder with agoraphobia by integrating local neural information. JAMA Psychiatry 2015;72:68–74.

45. Ma N, Li L, Shu N, et al. White matter abnormalities in first-episode, treatment-naive young adults with major depressive disorder. Am J Psychiatry 2007;164:823–6.

46. Martinez D, Carpenter KM, Liu F, et al. Imaging dopamine transmission in cocaine dependence: link between neurochemistry and response to treatment. Am J Psychiatry 2011;168:634–41.

47. Whitfield-Gabrieli S, Ghosh SS, Nieto-Castanon A, et al. Brain connectomics predict response to treatment in social anxiety disorder. Mol Psychiatry 2016;21:680–5.

48. Li F, Lui S, Yao L, et al. Longitudinal changes in resting-state cerebral activity in patients with first-episode schizophrenia: a 1-year follow-up functional MR imaging study. Radiology 2016;279:867–75.

49. Addington J, Heinssen R. Prediction and prevention of psychosis in youth at clinical high risk. Annu Rev Clin Psychol 2012;8:269–89.

50. Beardslee WR, Brent DA, Weersing VR, et al. Prevention of depression in at-risk adolescents: longer-term effects. JAMA Psychiatry 2013;70:1161–70.

51. Cao H, Chen OY, Chung Y, et al. Cerebello-thalamo-cortical hyperconnectivity as a state-independent functional neural signature for psychosis prediction and characterization. Nat Commun 2018;9:3836.

52. Chung Y, Addington J, Bearden CE, et al. Use of machine learning to determine deviance in neuro-anatomical maturity associated with future psychosis in youths at clinically high risk. JAMA Psychiatry 2018;75:960–8.

53. Krueger G, Granziera C, Jack CR Jr, et al. Effects of MRI scan acceleration on brain volume measurement consistency. J Magn Reson Imaging 2012;36:1234–40.

54. Caramanos Z, Fonov VS, Francis SJ, et al. Gradient distortions in MRI: characterizing and correcting for their effects on SIENA-generated measures of brain volume change. Neuroimage 2010;49:1601–11.

55. Preboske GM, Gunter JL, Ward CP, et al. Common MRI acquisition non-idealities significantly impact the output of the boundary shift integral method of measuring brain atrophy on serial MRI. Neuroimage 2006;30:1196–202.

56. Zhang F, Chen G, He M, et al. Altered white matter microarchitecture in amyotrophic lateral sclerosis: a voxel-based meta-analysis of diffusion tensor imaging. Neuroimage Clin 2018;19:122–9.

57. Chen G, Hu X, Li L, et al. Disorganization of white matter architecture in major depressive disorder: a meta-analysis of diffusion tensor imaging with tract-based spatial statistics. Sci Rep 2016;6:21825.

58. Church JA, Petersen SE, Schlaggar BL. The "Task B problem" and other considerations in developmental functional neuroimaging. Hum Brain Mapp 2010;31:852–62.

59. Kruggel F, Turner J, Muftuler LT, et al. Impact of scanner hardware and imaging protocol on image quality and compartment volume precision in the ADNI cohort. Neuroimage 2010;49:2123–33.

60. Manoach DS, Halpern EF, Kramer TS, et al. Test-retest reliability of a functional MRI working memory paradigm in normal and schizophrenic subjects. Am J Psychiatry 2001;158:955–8.

61. Zhao N, Yuan LX, Jia XZ, et al. Intra- and inter-scanner reliability of voxel-wise whole-brain analytic metrics for resting state fMRI. Front Neuroinform 2018;12:54.

62. Jovicich J, Czanner S, Han X, et al. MRI-derived measurements of human subcortical, ventricular and intracranial brain volumes: reliability effects of scan sessions, acquisition sequences, data analyses, scanner upgrade, scanner vendors and field strengths. Neuroimage 2009;46:177–92.

63. Lee H, Nakamura K, Narayanan S, et al. Estimating and accounting for the effect of MRI scanner changes on longitudinal whole-brain volume change measurements. Neuroimage 2019;184:555–65.

64. Khalili-Mahani N, Rombouts SARB, van Osch MJP, et al. Biomarkers, designs, and interpretations of resting-state fMRI in translational pharmacological

research: a review of state-of-the-Art, challenges, and opportunities for studying brain chemistry. Hum Brain Mapp 2017;38:2276–325.

65. Bocchetta M, Boccardi M, Ganzola R, et al. Harmonized benchmark labels of the hippocampus on magnetic resonance: the EADC-ADNI project. Alzheimers Dement 2015;11:151–60.e5.

66. Pearlson G. Multisite collaborations and large databases in psychiatric neuroimaging: advantages, problems, and challenges. Schizophr Bull 2009; 35:1–2.

67. Ma Q, Zhang T, Zanetti MV, et al. Classification of multi-site MR images in the presence of heterogeneity using multi-task learning. Neuroimage Clin 2018;19:476–86.

68. Wang X, Zhang T, Chaim TM, et al. Classification of MRI under the presence of disease heterogeneity using multi-task learning: application to bipolar disorder. Med Image Comput Comput Assist Interv 2015;9349:125–32.

69. Stevens JR. An anatomy of Schizophrenia? Arch Gen Psychiatry 1973;29:177.

70. Rozycki M, Satterthwaite TD, Koutsouleris N, et al. Multisite machine learning analysis provides a robust structural imaging signature of schizophrenia detectable across diverse patient populations and within individuals. Schizophr Bull 2018; 44:1035–44.

71. Scarpazza C, De Simone M. Voxel-based morphometry: current perspectives. Neurosci Neuroecon 2016;5:19–35.

72. Salvador R, Radua J, Canales-Rodriguez EJ, et al. Evaluation of machine learning algorithms and structural features for optimal MRI-based diagnostic prediction in psychosis. PLoS One 2017; 12:e0175683.

73. Steele VR, Rao V, Calhoun VD, et al. Machine learning of structural magnetic resonance imaging predicts psychopathic traits in adolescent offenders. Neuroimage 2017;145:265–73.

74. Zhang J, Liu W, Zhang J, et al. Distinguishing adolescents with conduct disorder from typically developing youngsters based on pattern classification of brain structural MRI. Front Hum Neurosci 2018;12:152.

75. Wang D, Li M, Wang M, et al. Individual-specific functional connectivity markers track dimensional and categorical features of psychotic illness. Mol Psychiatry 2018. https://doi.org/10.1038/s41380-018-0276-1.

76. Huang X, Gong Q, Sweeney JA, et al. Progress in psychoradiology, the clinical application of psychiatric neuroimaging. Br J Radiol 2019;92(1101): 20181000.

77. Abi-Dargham A, Horga G. The search for imaging biomarkers in psychiatric disorders. Nat Med 2016;22:1248–55.

78. Glasser MF, Sotiropoulos SN, Wilson JA, et al. The minimal preprocessing pipelines for the Human Connectome Project. Neuroimage 2013;80: 105–24.

79. Kempton MJ, McGuire P. How can neuroimaging facilitate the diagnosis and stratification of patients with psychosis? Eur Neuropsychopharmacol 2015; 25:725–32.

80. Smieskova R, Allen P, Simon A, et al. Different duration of at-risk mental state associated with neurofunctional abnormalities. A multimodal imaging study. Hum Brain Mapp 2012;33:2281–94.

81. Fusar-Poli P, Howes OD, Allen P, et al. Abnormal frontostriatal interactions in people with prodromal signs of psychosis: a multimodal imaging study. Arch Gen Psychiatry 2010;67:683–91.

82. Radua J, Borgwardt S, Crescini A, et al. Multimodal meta-analysis of structural and functional brain changes in first episode psychosis and the effects of antipsychotic medication. Neurosci Biobehav Rev 2012;36:2325–33.

83. Xiang L, Chen Y, Chang W, et al. Deep leaning based multi-modal fusion for fast MR reconstruction. IEEE Trans Biomed Eng 2019;66(7):2105–14.

84. Jauhar S, McCutcheon R, Borgan F, et al. The relationship between cortical glutamate and striatal dopamine in first-episode psychosis: a cross-sectional multimodal PET and magnetic resonance spectroscopy imaging study. Lancet Psychiatry 2018;5:816–23.

85. Howes O, McCutcheon R, Stone J. Glutamate and dopamine in schizophrenia: an update for the 21st century. J Psychopharmacol 2015;29:97–115.

86. Schifani C, Hafizi S, Da Silva T, et al. Using molecular imaging to understand early schizophrenia-related psychosis neurochemistry: a review of human studies. Int Rev Psychiatry 2017;29:555–66.

87. Salavati B, Rajji TK, Price R, et al. Imaging-based neurochemistry in schizophrenia: a systematic review and implications for dysfunctional long-term potentiation. Schizophr Bull 2014;41:44–56.

88. Vernon AC, Crum WR, Lerch JP, et al. Reduced cortical volume and elevated astrocyte density in rats chronically treated with antipsychotic drugs-linking magnetic resonance imaging findings to cellular pathology. Biol Psychiatry 2014; 75:982–90.

89. Vernon AC, Natesan S, Modo M, et al. Effect of chronic antipsychotic treatment on brain structure: a serial magnetic resonance imaging study with ex vivo and postmortem confirmation. Biol Psychiatry 2011;69:936–44.

90. Dorph-Petersen KA, Lewis DA. Postmortem structural studies of the thalamus in schizophrenia. Schizophr Res 2017;180:28–35.

91. Erp TGMV, Hibar DP, Rasmussen JM, et al. Subcortical brain volume abnormalities in 2028 individuals

with schizophrenia and 2540 healthy controls via the ENIGMA consortium. Mol Psychiatry 2016;21: 547–53.

92. Shepherd AM, Laurens KR, Matheson SL, et al. Systematic meta-review and quality assessment of the structural brain alterations in schizophrenia. Neurosci Biobehav Rev 2012;36:1342–56.

93. Couture SM, Penn DL, Losh M, et al. Comparison of social cognitive functioning in schizophrenia and high functioning autism: more convergence than divergence. Psychol Med 2010;40:569–79.

94. Hommer RE, Swedo SE. Schizophrenia and autism-related disorders. Schizophr Bull 2015;41: 313–4.

95. Pina-Camacho L, Parellada M, Kyriakopoulos M. Autism spectrum disorder and schizophrenia: boundaries and uncertainties. BJPsych Adv 2016; 22:316–24.

96. Ivleva EI, Clementz BA, Dutcher AM, et al. Brain structure biomarkers in the psychosis biotypes: findings from the bipolar-schizophrenia network for intermediate phenotypes. Biol Psychiatry 2017;82:26–39.

97. Hill SK, Reilly JL, Keefe RS, et al. Neuropsychological impairments in schizophrenia and psychotic bipolar disorder: findings from the Bipolar-Schizophrenia Network on Intermediate Phenotypes (B-SNIP) study. Am J Psychiatry 2013;170: 1275–84.

98. Wang JB, Zheng LJ, Cao QJ, et al. Inconsistency in abnormal brain activity across cohorts of ADHD-200 in children with attention deficit hyperactivity disorder. Front Neurosci 2017;11:320.

99. Consortium H. The ADHD-200 consortium: a model to advance the translational potential of neuroimaging in clinical neuroscience. Front Syst Neurosci 2012;6:62.

100. Skatun KC, Kaufmann T, Doan NT, et al. Consistent functional connectivity alterations in schizophrenia spectrum disorder: a multisite study. Schizophr Bull 2017;43:914–24.

Resting-State Functional Connectivity: Signal Origins and Analytic Methods

Kai Chen, PhD[a], Azeezat Azeez, PhD[b], Donna Y. Chen, BE[b],
Bharat B. Biswal, PhD[a,b],*

KEYWORDS

- Functional MRI • BOLD signal • Resting-state functional connectivity • Psychoradiology
- Functional connectivity • Brain connectivity • Resting state

KEY POINTS

- Resting State Functional MRI (fMRI) has evolved into a method for mapping brain function in healthy and clinical neuroimaging.
- Resting State fMRI can be used to map brain function instead of task activation where the subject has to perform a task.
- Resting-state functional connectivity (RSFC) may be defined as a significant temporal correlation between functionally related brain regions in the absence of any stimulus or task.

INTRODUCTION

Because of its high spatial and temporal resolution in addition to its noninvasiveness, functional MRI (fMRI) has become the method of choice for studying systems-level brain function. fMRI uses the BOLD (blood-oxygen-level-dependent) signal, discovered by Seiji Ogawa in 1991. It is currently understood that task activation or stimulus presentation leads to an increase in neuronal firing in the eloquent regions of the brain. Increased neuronal firing leads to increased oxygen consumption and vasodilation. The activation-induced increase in brain oxygenation reduces intravascular deoxyhemoglobin and therefore decreases susceptibility-induced intravoxel dephasing. Spin coherence increases, resulting in increased signal intensity. Brain activation is observed as localized signal enhancement. Activity in voxels and coherence of that activity with activity in other regions are widely used indices of brain activity and functional connectivity respectively. These measures are informative and widely used tools for assessing brain function, contributing to psychoradiology, a subspecialty of radiology first described by Lui and colleagues,[1] devoted to translating psychiatric imaging research to advance diagnostic and therapeutic practice in clinical psychiatry.

TASK-ACTIVATION DESIGN

Brain mapping experiment typically consists of alternating periods of stimulus task and control state and the cycle is repeated several times. Images are collected throughout the cycles and the

Funding: Dr B. Biswal has received funding from NIH R01AT009829 for this article.
[a] The Clinical Hospital of Chengdu Brain Science Institute, MOE Key Laboratory for Neuroinformation, Center for Information in Medicine, School of Life Science and Technology, University of Electronic Science and Technology of China, No.2006, Xiyuan Avenue, West Hi-Tech Zone, Chengdu, Sichuan 611731, China; [b] Department of Biomedical Engineering, New Jersey Institute of Technology, 619 Fenster Hall, Newark, NJ 07102, USA
* Corresponding author. The Clinical Hospital of Chengdu Brain Science Institute, MOE Key Laboratory for Neuroinformation, Center for Information in Medicine, School of Life Science and Technology, University of Electronic Science and Technology of China, No.2006, Xiyuan Avenue, West Hi-Tech Zone, Chengdu, Sichuan 611731, China.
E-mail address: bbiswal@gmail.com

image acquisition is repeated at several intervals of the time of repetition (TR) throughout the experiment, while the subject alternates between the stimulus and control task. It is typically assumed that the magnitude of the BOLD effect reflects the magnitude of the neural activity change. A standard method of task presentation uses a box-car or block design where blocks of the stimulus or task are presented typically for 20-30 seconds, alternating with periods of rest or a control condition. By subtracting the brain regions recruited during the performance of the control task from the brain regions recruited during the test condition, the areas of the brain whose activity is associated specifically with the cognitive process of interest can be identified.

- The activation-induced increase in brain oxygenation reduces intravascular deoxyhemoglobin and thus decreases susceptibility-induced intravoxel dephasing.

RESTING-STATE FUNCTIONAL CONNECTIVITY

Resting-state functional connectivity (RSFC) may be defined as significant temporal correlation between functionally related brain regions in the absence of any stimulus or task. The authors' group[2] first demonstrated a significant temporal correlation of spontaneous low-frequency signal fluctuations (SLFs) both within and across hemispheres in primary sensorimotor cortex during rest. Voxels from the sensorimotor region and its associated cortices correlated significantly (after filtering the fundamental and harmonics of respiration and heart rates), whereas only a few voxel time courses (<3%) correlated with those in regions outside the motor cortex. This correlated signal arises from SLFs. In 1997, Lowe and colleagues[3] extended the results of Biswal and colleagues[2] by showing such correlations over larger regions of the sensorimotor cortex (ie, across multiple slices).

Subsequently, in 2002 Hampson and colleagues[4] demonstrated the presence of RSFC in sensory cortices, specifically auditory and visual cortex. In their studies, a signal from visual cortex voxels during rest (first scan) was used as a reference and correlated with every other voxel in the brain. A significant number of voxels from the visual cortex passed a threshold of 0.35, whereas only a few voxels from outside the visual cortex passed the threshold. These investigators produced similar results in the auditory cortex.[5]

Xiong and colleagues[6-8] established relationships between motor and association cortices. Similar to earlier studies, they observed resting-state connectivity between sensorimotor cortex areas (primary, premotor, secondary somatosensory) as well as RSFC relationships between these motor areas and association areas, specifically anterior and posterior cingulate cortex, regions known to be involved in attention. Greicius and colleagues[9] observed resting-state connectivity in anterior and posterior cingulate areas. Subsequent observation of activation during a visual attention task indicated similar cingulate activity.

These studies have established the foundation for "resting-state functional connectivity studies" using fMRI (eg, Refs.[2–4,9,10]). Results from these studies form the basis for speculation regarding the functional role of resting-state connectivity. Bressler[11] has suggested that such correlated SLFs may be a phenomenon representing the functional connection of cortical areas analogous to the phenomenon of "effective connectivity," defined by Friston and colleagues[12] as the temporal connectivity between brain regions in response to tasks.

Biophysical-Origin Hypotheses of Resting-State Functional Connectivity

The role of SLFs and, consequently, RSFC and its biophysiologic origin have not been completely understood. Cooper and colleagues[13] hypothesized that these fluctuations represent cellular maintenance of an optimum balance between blood flow and cerebral metabolic rate. Testing this hypothesis has involved manipulation of cerebral metabolism with anesthesia. These studies have involved comparison of activity during waking and anesthetized states in animals using various techniques including laser Doppler flowmetry (LDF)[14] and fMRI in humans.[15,16] Signal oscillations in the rodent brain vary with differing levels of halothane anesthesia, Pco_2, and nitric oxide synthase blockade LDF.[14] These results suggest support for the biophysical-origin hypothesis that affects the neural vasculature. The neural mechanisms of slow rhythmic fluctuations have not yet been clearly defined, although studies indicate that they may be both neuronal and glial in origin.[17]

Using MR echo-planar imaging, the authors have previously investigated whether respiratory hypercapnia, which is known to suspend spontaneous oscillations in regional cerebral blood flow, influences these low-frequency fluctuations.[18] The magnitude of low-frequency fluctuations was reversibly diminished during hypercapnia, resulting in a substantial decrease of the temporal correlation both within and across contralateral hemispheres of the sensorimotor cortex. After the breathing gas mixture was replaced by room air, the magnitude and spatial extent of the temporal correlation of low-frequency fluctuations returned to normal. Results of this study support the hypothesis that low-frequency physiologic fluctuations observed by MR in the human cortex and spontaneous flow oscillations observed in early studies by LDF in the cortex of the rat are identical and are secondary to fluctuations in neuronal activity.

In a recent study, Mateo and colleagues[19] provided important evidence from studies on mouse cortex during modulation of vasomotion, that is, intrinsic ultraslow (0.1 Hz) fluctuations in arteriole diameter. They demonstrated that the natural ~0.1-Hz oscillatory dilations and constrictions of arterioles phase lock to ultraslow variations in the envelope of the high-frequency electrical activity in cortex, that is, γ-band power. Furthermore, this occurred under resting-state conditions and in response to the optogenetic drive of the cortex. This further suggests that the RSFC has a neuronal mechanism.

Cognitive-Origin Hypotheses of Resting-State Functional Connectivity

In contrast to the biophysical-origin hypotheses, others have proposed cognitive-origin hypotheses, based on observations that low-frequency SLFs appear to correlate between functionally connected brain areas (eg, Refs.[20,21]). Testing these hypotheses has involved observation of resting-state activity between functionally connected regions, and contrasts in between. Thus, a family of cognitive-origin hypotheses (in contrast to biophysical-origin hypotheses) has emerged. Gusnard and colleagues,[10] for instance, have suggested that such coherence indicates the presence of a "default mode of brain function" whereby a default network continuously monitors external (eg, visual stimuli) and internal (eg, body-functions, emotions) stimuli. Other cognitive-origin hypotheses suggest that low-frequency fluctuation is related to ongoing problem-solving and planning.[9] Biswal and colleagues[2] and Xiong and colleagues[6,7] observed that analyses of resting-state physiologic fluctuations reveal many more functional connections than those revealed by task-induced activation analysis. They hypothesized that task-induced activation maps underestimate the size and number of functionally connected areas and that functional networks are more fully revealed by RSFC analysis. This is in accordance with the psychoradiology hypothesis by Gong and colleagues, who proposed a "brain structure-function-

behavioral conjunction" theory in which brain structural alteration leads to clinical syndromes via impact on widely distributed functional connectivity.[1,22–25] Of note, Gong's psychoradiology theory sets milestone from the perspective of translational psychiatric imaging, and it leads to a series of discoveries of the imaging biomarkers specific to a variety of psychiatric disorders.

Resting-State Functional Connectivity Data Analysis

A great number of methods to analyze resting-state fMRI data exist. Because recent reviews have described these methods in detail,[26,27] they are only briefly described here. The analysis methods can be described in terms of time domain or frequency domain. Analysis performed in the time domain uses temporal properties of the signal to estimate the parameters, whereas frequency-domain methods estimate the frequencies of significance.

Time-domain analysis

Seed-based correlation is one of the oldest and simplest measures of functional connectivity[2] and assumes that if 2 or more regions (or voxels) are functionally related, they will be temporally correlated. In this method, the user selects a region (or voxel) and the corresponding time series is then correlated with every other region (or voxels) in the brain, and a connectivity map is then estimated. A limitation of this method lies in the fact that a priori information regarding the selection of the seed region is essential.

Regional homogeneity estimates the connectivity of voxels with its neighboring voxels, using Kendall's correlation statistic. This method was proposed by Zang and colleagues[8] in 2004, and assumes that a given voxel that is significantly correlated with many of its neighboring voxels is more functionally connected. Numerically, the time series of one voxel is correlated with its immediate neighbors, and this is performed simultaneously for each voxel. The spatial extent of its neighbors can be defined by the cluster size, typically 27 voxels. Kendall's correlation coefficient is used to measure the correlation between a given voxel and its neighbors. A whole brain map is created showing underlying connectivity activations of clusters.

Principal and independent component analysis involves multivariate data-driven analysis methods that reduce large multidimensional data sets into a reduced number of components that capture most of the information of the original data sets. In principal component analysis (PCA), the first component captures the maximum variability of the overall signal and the second component, which is orthogonal to the first, captures the maximum variability of the residual signal. This is repeated until most of the variability of the original signal can be accounted for. These components and, consequently, networks are produced without any prior assumptions. Limitations of PCA are that orthogonality of the components does not necessitate independence, and thus a signal of interest may be misrepresented.[28] To circumvent some of these issues, independent component analysis (ICA), a data-driven approach that looks for the existence of statistically independent spatial-temporal maps across the brain, is used. PCA is the precursor to ICA because this approach extracts the common component across the data; unlike ICA, it does not assume Gaussian distribution.[29] One of the major challenges in ICA is the assignment of spatial maps corresponding to brain function.

Frequency-domain methods

Amplitude of low frequency fluctuations (ALFF) assumes that the relevant information in the BOLD signal giving rise to RSFC is below 0.1 Hz and can be represented by a single parameter. First described by Zou, Zuo and colleagues,[30,31] this parameter is calculated by averaging the square root of the power of low-frequency BOLD signals and standardizing the values to a global mean ALFF value. ALFF can be influenced by background noise, and a high value can be produced around vasculature and the edges of the brain. To account for some of the limitations of ALFF, a more refined technique, known as fractional ALLF (fALLF), has been developed. fALFF is defined as the ratio of the power at each frequency to the integrated power of the entire frequency range across the frequency of interest, in the 0.01- to 0.1-Hz range, then dividing by the amplitude sum across the entire range.

Coherence analysis is the spectral representation of the correlation in the frequency domain.[32] It is defined as the square of the cross-spectrum over the product of one time-series power spectrum times the other. This allows for the study of time course, as known artifacts can be easily filtered from the data.

COMPARISONS OF RESTING-STATE FUNCTIONAL CONNECTIVITY AND TASK-INDUCED ACTIVITY

Skudlarski and Gore[33] compared RSFC and SLFs in the olfactory cortex during 3 sustained passive stimuli: a pleasant odor, an unpleasant odor, and no odor. They reported that the presentation of odor altered the strength of correlation in some regions in comparison with the rest. Biswal and Hyde[34] studied low-frequency physiologic fluctuations in the motor cortex during a sustained 6-min period of bilateral finger tapping. In all 4 subjects, the frequency and phase of low-frequency fluctuations was similar. The magnitude of the low-frequency fluctuations, however, was significantly enhanced during continuous finger tapping. In addition, RSFC maps produced by correlation of low-frequency fluctuations between motor-cortex voxels had an improved coincidence with task-activation maps compared with RSFC. These 3 studies involved a sustained active task or a sustained change in environment, or a sustained task that was repeated twice with different instructions. Numerous other variants and extensions of these ideas are immediately apparent. However, in each case one is comparing differences between small effects. There is a significant challenge to improve experimental methodologies for these kinds of experiments.

The results of these studies suggest intriguing clues about the relationship between RSFC, functional activity, and the role of attention in mediating these relationships. Thus, Gusnard and colleagues,[10] for instance, have argued that the set of brain regions showing correlated activity at rest (the "default" network) continuously monitors external (eg, visual stimuli) and internal (eg, body functions, emotions) stimuli. Based on similar observations, and apparent hippocampal involvement, Greicius and colleagues[9] have argued that RSFC may be related to episodic memory retrieval in the service of ongoing problem-solving and planning. Moreover, such activity may be suppressed or "suspended"[10] under conditions of demanding cognitive activity. Such accounts are intriguing because they suggest that presumed baseline activity may not be as random as has been nearly universally presumed. Others have argued that RSFC represents the tonic activation of networks that are brought "on line" during cognitive task performance. All of these hypotheses suggest that meaningful functional activity may be occurring during rest. Understanding the mechanisms and the functional and clinical relevance of such activity may have profound effects on our understanding of functional neuroimaging results, leading to explanations, for example, of many poorly understood "negative correlations."

The authors and others have investigated meta-analytic coactivation patterns among brain regions based on published neuroimaging studies, and have compared the coactivation network configurations with those in the resting-state network.[35,36] The strength of RSFC between 2 regions was strongly correlated with the coactivation strength.

However, the coactivation network showed greater global efficiency, smaller mean clustering coefficient, and lower modularity compared with the resting-state network, which suggests a more efficient global information transmission and between-system integrations during task performance. Changes in network properties were also observed within the thalamus and the left inferior temporal cortex. The thalamus and the left inferior temporal cortex exhibited higher and lower degrees, respectively, in the coactivation network compared with the resting-state network. These results shed light regarding the reconfiguration of the brain networks between task and resting-state conditions, and highlight the role of the thalamus in the change of network configurations in task versus rest.

APPLICATION TO AGING

Furthermore, understanding RSFC-activation relationships could also lead to plausible accounts for patterns in age-related differences in BOLD activity (eg, Refs.[37–42]) because older adults often show greater activation than younger counterparts. Cognitive accounts of this phenomenon, such as "age-related compensation," have been unsatisfactory thus far because age-related activation increases have not been consistently related to performance improvements in older adults (eg, Refs.[37,39]). The idea that such age-related activation increases are related to an RSFC network that must be inhibited for successful task performance is compelling because older adults are known to have deficits in inhibitory functions at the cellular (ie, neuronal), structural (ie, glial), and cognitive (ie, behavioral[43]) levels. Greicius and colleagues,[9] however, have observed decreased hippocampal involvement in comparisons between older healthy and Alzheimer's disease patients.

Task-related patterns of BOLD activity may represent acute activation of the circuits necessary for the task at hand. Such circuitry may be revealed in effective connectivity analysis models advanced by several researchers (eg, Refs.[44–46]). These analyses have revealed interconnections between brain regions known to be active during cognitive task performance. In one working memory study, for instance, McIntosh and colleagues[46] observed increases in interactions among prefrontal cortex (PFC) regions and between PFC and corticolimbic regions with increasing delay intervals. Effective connectivity studies comparing younger and older adults have indicated that older adults show increased connectivity during cognitive task performance.

Their results indicated that, whereas younger adults showed hippocampal interactions with ventral PFC during memory encoding, older adults show hippocampal interactions with both dorsal and ventral as well as parietal interactions. At present, the meaning of this age-related and disease-related increased connectivity remains poorly understood. The best evidence suggests that it may reflect either (1) compensatory activity in the service of optimizing memory performance[37] or (2) a decreased inhibition of the "default mode," as Greicius and colleagues[9] have suggested. Little leverage may be gained from these questions because the results come from different groups of subjects performing different tasks.

Neuropsychological and functional neuroimaging studies indicate that attention is subserved by anatomically overlapping but functionally dissociable networks in the brain.[47] A posterior network that includes the superior parietal lobe and its connections to inferior temporal and lateral premotor regions is important for voluntary detection of target stimuli in space (termed selective attention[48]). An anterior network that includes the anterior cingulate and its connections to dorsolateral prefrontal cortex is important for monitoring target detection and for maintaining target-related and goal-related information in working memory while resisting interference from competing information (termed executive control). The parietal and frontal cortices are anatomically connected directly as well as indirectly via the anterior cingulate gyrus. The anatomic connectivity facilitates goal-directed behavior that is accomplished by continuous interaction of operations of selective attention and executive control.

Life-span development seems to reflect disproportionate changes in anterior attentional networks. Cognitive development from childhood into adulthood includes improved executive control of action and attention. These cognitive improvements are subserved by functional anatomic maturation of the prefrontal cortex and associated anterior cingulate circuitry.[41,49] Conversely, normal aging is marked by declines in executive control that are related to reductions in inhibitory functions (eg, Hasher and colleagues[43]) and functional changes in prefrontal cortex and associated circuitry.[38,42] These findings suggest that the anterior attentional network may be relatively more affected by the deleterious effects of adult aging, and that anterior rather than posterior attentional networks are more influenced by neural changes associated with childhood development and aging.

Evidence suggests that whereas the anterior attentional network is disproportionately affected by diseases of childhood, diseases of aging may affect both anterior and posterior attention networks (eg, Vaidya and colleagues[50]). Clinically, attention-deficit hyperactivity disorder (ADHD) is characterized by impulsivity, inattention, and hyperactivity. In the laboratory it is characterized by reductions in performance on anterior attention tasks (eg, "go/no-go" and "n-back"[51]) but relatively preserved performance on visual search tasks.[27,52] Patients with Alzheimer disease, on the other hand, tend to show deficits in both kinds of tasks.[53–55]

CHALLENGES AND LIMITATIONS

Because of its simplicity, RSFC has become a popular method to study brain function, especially in clinical settings where the subjects cannot perform certain tasks. As a result, the clinical applicability of resting-state fMRI is rapidly expanding. Thus, there is a need to address and overcome limitations of resting-state methods.

Even a small amount of head motion can result in BOLD signal distortions that can affect the various connectivity measures. The impact of head movement on RSFC measures has been documented in pediatric, adolescent, and aging populations, where the magnitude of micromovement has been associated with diminished long-range connections and increased short-range connections such as in the homologous primary motor cortex.[56–59] Subject-level motion correction seems to be inadequate in efficiently removing individual-specific motion effects. Hence, additional steps of correction such as mean framewise displacement have been recommended at group-level analysis.

The average time series from the whole brain, comprising both the gray matter and white matter, is typically regressed from all of the voxels.[60] Although the global average time series is expected to account for confounders such as head motion and other sources of physiologic noise, there is a major caveat. Several studies have shown that it tends to result in more negative correlations.[60] Furthermore, electrophysiologic studies in monkeys suggest a neuronal basis to the average global signal.[61,62] Therefore, especially in clinical populations, removing the average global signal may carry information corresponding to the subject and risk the removal of true neuronal effects. A lack of consensus on a one-way fix-all approach to remove noise in resting-state fMRI data emphasizes the need for careful design of preprocessing and postprocessing strategies depending on the specific goals and population studied.

Methodologic limitations exist in resting-state metrics, which calls for an urgent need to address and overcome these limitations to achieve high test-retest reliability. At present, low intraindividual and high interindividual variability in resting-state connectivity metrics establishes the stability and selectivity necessary for developing clinical tests, with the use of neuroimaging biomarkers. Most resting-state data-processing strategies result in fair to high reliability depending on the different RSFC parameters used.[63,64] Simple measures such as scanning in a fixed resting-state setting can improve reliability. For instance, studies show that a scan duration of just 5 minutes is sufficient for 50% reliability, whereas increasing the duration to 13 minutes for intrasession and 9 minutes for intersession has been shown to further improve reliability. However, many of the reliability issues arise from physiologic noise and preprocessing procedures.[65,66]

SUMMARY

Despite some methodologic limitations, resting-state fMRI holds great promise for the translation of neuroimaging findings to clinical application. For instance, it provides potentially useful functional biomarkers for psychiatric subtyping, and for the first time, Drysdale and colleagues defined depression subtypes in individual patients although Sun and colleagues were the first to subtype psychiatric disorders based on structural imaging features using an unsupervised machine learning technique/algorithm.[67,68]

Resting-state fMRI technique inherently possesses the advantage of allowing the investigation of the brain's intrinsic activity with greater signal-to-noise ratio while also avoiding confounders associated with task.[69] The advancement of data analysis and noise-correction techniques has extended the application of resting-state fMRI to populations that were previously difficult to scan, such as neonates, the cognitively challenged, and those facing issues with sleep and sedation. Furthermore, high temporal resolution and multiband imaging technology have allowed studies to record meaningful spontaneous fluctuations at higher frequencies of up to 0.75 Hz. However, the functional implication of this has yet to be established[70-74] and, of course, combining resting-state data with other modalities could serve to bridge the gap between functional findings and other biomarkers for prediction, diagnosis, and prognosis of clinical conditions.[1,22,25,75–78] Nevertheless, more work is required to improve the reliability of multimodal studies before resting-state fMRI can be routinely and more widely used in the clinical realm.

REFERENCES

1. Lui S, Zhou XJ, Sweeney JA, et al. Psychoradiology: the frontier of neuroimaging in psychiatry. Radiology 2016;281:357–72.
2. Biswal B, Yetkin FZ, Haughton VM, et al. Functional connectivity in the motor cortex of resting human brain using echo-planar MRI. Magn Reson Med 1995;34. https://doi.org/10.1002/mrm.1910340409.
3. Lowe MJ, Rutecki P, Turski P, et al. Auditory cortex FMRI noise correlations in callosal agenesis. Neuroimage 1997;5:S194.
4. Hampson M, Peterson BS, Skuldarski P, et al. Changes in functional connectivity using temporal correlations in MR images. Hum Brain Mapp 2002; 15:247.
5. Hampson M, Olson IR, Leung HC, et al. Changes in functional connectivity of human MT/V5 with visual motion input. Neuroreport 2004;7:1315.
6. Xiong JP, Pu LM, Gao Y, et al. Improved interregional connectivity mapping by use of covariance analysis within rest condition. ISMRM Sixth Scientific Meeting & Exhibition. Sydney, Australia, April 18–24, 1998.
7. Xiong J, Parsons LM, Gao JH, et al. Interregional connectivity to primary motor cortex revealed using MRI resting state images. Hum Brain Mapp 1999; 8(2–3):151–6.
8. Zang Y, Jiang T, Lu Y, et al. Regional homogeneity approach to fMRI data analysis. Neuroimage 2004; 22(1):394–400.
9. Greicius MD, Srivastava G, Reiss AL, et al. Default-mode network activity distinguishes Alzheimer's disease from healthy aging: evidence from functional MRI. Proc Natl Acad Sci U S A 2004;101(13): 4637–42.
10. Gusnard DA, Raichle ME. Searching for a baseline: functional imaging and the resting human brain. Nat Rev Neurosci 2001;10:685–94.
11. Bressler S. Large-scale cortical networks and cognition. Brain Res Brain Res Rev 1996;20:288–304.
12. Friston KJ, Frith CD, Liddle PF, et al. Functional connectivity: the principal component analysis of large (PET) data sets. J Cereb Blood Flow Metab 1993; 13:5.
13. Cooper R, Crow HJ, Walter WG, et al. Regional control of cerebral vascular reactivity and oxygen supply in man. Brain Res 1966;3:174.
14. Hudetz AG, Roman RJ, Harder DR. Spontaneous flow oscillations in the cerebral cortex during acute changes in mean arterial pressure. J Cereb Blood Flow Metab 1992;12:491.
15. Biswal B, Bandettini PA, Jesmanowicz A, et al. Time-frequency analysis of functional EPI time-course series. SMRM Twelfth Annual Scientific Meeting. New York, August 14–20, 1993.
16. Weisskoff RM, Baker J, Belliveau J, et al. Poser spectrum analysis of functionally-weighted MR data: what's in the noise? SMRM Twelfth Annual Scientific Meeting. New York, August 14–20, 1993.
17. Zonta M, Angulo MC, Gobbo S, et al. Neuron-to-astrocyte signaling is central to the dynamic control of brain microcirculation. Nat Neurosci 2003;6: 43–50.
18. Biswal BB, Kannurpatti SS, Rypma B. Hemodynamic scaling of fMRI-BOLD signal: validation of low-frequency spectral amplitude as a scalability factor. Magn Reson Imaging 2007;25(10):1358–69.
19. Mateo C, Knutsen PM, Tsai PS, et al. Entrainment of arteriole vasomotor fluctuations by neural activity is a basis of blood-oxygenation-level-dependent "resting-state" connectivity. Neuron 2017;96(4). 936–948.e3.
20. Biswal BB, Van Kylen J, Hyde JS. Simultaneous assessment of flow and BOLD signals in resting-state functional connectivity maps. NMR Biomed 1997;10:165–70.
21. Biswal B, Hudetz AG, Yetkin FZ, et al. Hypercapnia reversibly suppresses low-frequency fluctuations in the human motor cortex during rest using echo-planar MRI. J Cereb Blood Flow Metab 1997;17:301.
22. Gong Q, Lui S, Sweeney JA. A selective review of cerebral abnormalities in patients with first-episode schizophrenia before and after treatment. Am J Psychiatry 2016;173:232–43.
23. Lui S, Deng W, Huang X, et al. Association of cerebral deficits with clinical symptoms in antipsychotic-naive first-episode schizophrenia: an optimized voxel-based morphometry and resting state functional connectivity study. Am J Psychiatry 2009;166(2):196–205.
24. Tregellas J. Connecting brain structure and function in schizophrenia. Am J Psychiatry 2009;166:134–6.
25. Huang X, Gong Q, Sweeney JA, et al. Progress in psychoradiology, the clinical application of psychiatric neuroimaging. Br J Radiol 2019;92(1101). 20181000.
26. Smitha KA, Akhil Raja K, Arun KM, et al. Resting state fMRI: a review on methods in resting state connectivity analysis and resting state networks. Neuroradiol J 2017;30(4):305–17.
27. Azeez AK, Biswal BB. A review of resting-state analysis methods. Neuroimaging Clin N Am 2017;27(4): 581–92.
28. Huettel SA, Song AW, McCarthy G. Functional magnetic resonance imaging, vol. 1. Sunderland (MA): Sinauer Associates; 2004.
29. Beckmann CF, DeLuca M, Devlin JT, et al. Investigations into resting-state connectivity using independent component analysis. Philos Trans R Soc Lond B Biol Sci 2005;360(1457):1001–13.

30. Zou QH, Zhu CZ, Yang Y, et al. An improved approach to detection of amplitude of low-frequency fluctuation (ALFF) for resting-state fMRI: fractional ALFF. J Neurosci Methods 2008; 172(1):137–41.

31. Zuo XN, Di Martino A, Kelly C, et al. The oscillating brain: complex and reliable. Neuroimage 2010; 49(2):1432–45.

32. Li K, Guo L, Nie J, et al. Review of methods for functional brain connectivity detection using fMRI. Comput Med Imaging Graph 2009;33(2):131–9.

33. Skudlarski P, Gore JC. Changes in the correlations in the FMRI physiological fluctuations may reveal functional connectivity within the brain. Neuroimage 1998;3:S600.

34. Biswal BB, Hyde JS. Functional connectivity during continuous task activation. ISMRM Sixth Scientific Meeting & Exhibition. Sydney, Australia, April 18–24, 1998. p. 2132.

35. Di X, Gohel S, Kim EH, et al. Task vs. rest-different network configurations between the coactivation and the resting-state brain networks. Front Hum Neurosci 2013;7:493.

36. Smith SM, Fox PT, Miller KL, et al. Correspondence of the brain's functional architecture during activation and rest. Proc Natl Acad Sci U S A 2009;106: 13040–5.

37. Grady CL, McIntosh AR, Horwitz B, et al. Age-related reductions in human recognition memory due to impaired encoding. Science 1995; 269(5221):218–21.

38. Rypma B, D'Esposito M. Isolating the neural mechanisms of age-related changes in human working memory. Nat Neurosci 2000;3:509–15.

39. Rypma B, Prabhakaran V, Desmond JE, et al. Age differences in prefrontal cortical activity in working memory. Psychol Aging 2001;16:371–84.

40. Satterthwaite TD, Elliott MA, Gerraty RT, et al. An improved framework for confound regression and filtering for control of motion artifact in the preprocessing of resting-state functional connectivity data. Neuroimage 2013;64:240–56.

41. Cabeza R. Hemispheric asymmetry reduction in older adults: the HAROLD model. Psychol Aging 2002;17:85–100.

42. Rypma B, Berger JS, Genova H, et al. Dissociating age-related changes in cognitive strategy and neural efficiency using event-related fMRI. Cortex 2005;41(4):582–94.

43. Hasher L, Stoltzfus ER, Zacks RT, et al. Age and inhibition. J Exp Psychol Learn Mem Cogn 1991;17:163–9.

44. Buchel C, Friston K. Assessing interactions among neuronal systems using functional neuroimaging. Neural Netw 2000;13:871–82.

45. Goebel R, Roebroeck A, Kim DS, et al. Investigating directed cortical interactions in time-resolved fMRI data using vector autoregressive modeling and Granger causality mapping. Magn Reson Imaging 2003;21:1251–61.

46. McIntosh AR, Rajah MN, Lobaugh NJ. Interactions of prefrontal cortex in relation to awareness in sensory learning. Science 1999;284:1531–3.

47. Posner MI, Petersen SE. The attention system of the human brain. Annu Rev Neurosci 1990;13:25–42.

48. Corbetta M, Shulman GL. Human cortical mechanisms of visual attention during orienting and search. Philos Trans R Soc Lond B Biol Sci 1998; 353:1353–62.

49. Bunge SA, Dudukovic NM, Thomason ME, et al. Immature frontal lobe contributions to cognitive control in children: evidence from fMRI. Neuron 2002; 33:301–11.

50. Vaidya CJ, Bunge SA, Dudukovic NM, et al. Altered neural substrates of cognitive control in childhood ADHD: evidence from functional magnetic resonance imaging. Am J Psychiatry 2005; 162:1605–13.

51. Vaidya CJ, Austin G, Kirkorian G, et al. Selective effects of methylphenidate in attention deficit hyperactivity disorder: a functional magnetic resonance study. Proc Natl Acad Sci U S A 1999;95: 14494–9.

52. Aman CJ, Roberts RJ, Pennington BF. A neuropsychological examination of the underlying deficit in attention deficit hyperactivity disorder: frontal lobe versus right parietal lobe theories. Dev Psychol 1998;34:956–69.

53. Backman L, Jones S, Berger AK, et al. Cognitive impairment in preclinical Alzheimer's disease: a meta-analysis. Neuropsychology 2005;19:520–31.

54. Drzezga A, Grimmer T, Peller M, et al. Impaired cross-modal inhibition in Alzheimer's Disease. PLoS Med 2005;2:288.

55. Rosler A, Mapstone M, Hays-Wicklund A, et al. The "zoom lens" of focal attention in visual search: changes in aging and Alzheimer's disease. Cortex 2005;41:512–9.

56. Power JD, Barnes KA, Snyder AZ, et al. Spurious but systematic correlations in functional connectivity MRI networks arise from subject motion. Neuroimage 2012;59(3):2142–54.

57. Power JD, Mitra A, Laumann TO, et al. Methods to detect, characterize, and remove motion artifact in resting state fMRI. Neuroimage 2014;84:320–41.

58. Van Dijk KR, Sabuncu MR, Buckner RL. The influence of head motion on intrinsic functional connectivity MRI. Neuroimage 2012;59(1):431–8.

59. Satterthwaite TD, Wolf DH, Ruparel K, et al. Heterogeneous impact of motion on fundamental patterns of developmental changes in functional connectivity during youth. Neuroimage 2013;83:45–57.

60. Murphy K, Fox MD. Towards a consensus regarding global signal regression for resting state functional connectivity MRI. Neuroimage 2017;154:169–73.

61. Scholvinck ML, Maier A, Ye FQ, et al. Neural basis of global resting-state fMRI activity. Proc Natl Acad Sci U S A 2010;107(22):10238–43.

62. Wen H, Liu Z. Broadband electrophysiological dynamics contribute to global resting-state fMRI signal. J Neurosci 2016;36(22):6030–40.

63. Han Y, Wang J, Zhao Z, et al. Frequency-dependent changes in the amplitude of low-frequency fluctuations in amnestic mild cognitive impairment: a resting-state fMRI study. Neuroimage 2011;55(1): 287–95.

64. Zuo XN, Anderson JS, Bellec P, et al. An open science resource for establishing reliability and reproducibility in functional connectomics. Sci Data 2014;1:140049.

65. Birn RM, Molloy EK, Patriat R, et al. The effect of scan length on the reliability of resting-state fMRI connectivity estimates. Neuroimage 2013;83:550–8.

66. Van Dijk KR, Hedden T, Venkataraman A, et al. Intrinsic functional connectivity as a tool for human connectomics: theory, properties, and optimization. J Neurophysiol 2010;103(1):297–321.

67. Drysdale AT, Grosenick L, Downar J, et al. Resting-state connectivity biomarkers define neurophysiological subtypes of depression. Nat Med 2017; 23(1):28–38.

68. Sun H, Lui S, Yao L, et al. Two patterns of white matter abnormalities in medication-naive patients with first-episode schizophrenia revealed by diffusion tensor imaging and cluster analysis. JAMA Psychiatry 2015;72(7):678–86.

69. Fox MD, Greicius M. Clinical applications of resting state functional connectivity. Front Syst Neurosci 2010;4:19.

70. Boubela RN, Kalcher K, Huf W, et al. Beyond noise: using temporal ICA to extract meaningful information from high-frequency fMRI signal fluctuations during rest. Front Hum Neurosci 2013;7:168.

71. Cordes D, Haughton VM, Arfanakis K, et al. Frequencies contributing to functional connectivity in the cerebral cortex in "resting-state" data. AJNR Am J Neuroradiol 2001;22(7):1326–33.

72. Gohel SR, Biswal BB. Functional integration between brain regions at rest occurs in multiple-frequency bands. Brain Connect 2015; 5(1):23–34.

73. Lee H-L, Zahneisen B, Hugger T, et al. Tracking dynamic resting-state networks at higher frequencies using MR-encephalography. Neuroimage 2013;65: 216–22.

74. Wu CW, Gu H, Lu H, et al. Frequency specificity of functional connectivity in brain networks. Neuroimage 2008;42(3):1047–55.

75. Gong Q, Response to Sarpal, et al. Importance of neuroimaging biomarkers for treatment development and clinical practice. Am J Psychiatry 2016; 173:733–4.

76. Kressel HY. Setting Sail 2017. Radiology 2017; 282(1):4–6.

77. Port JD. Diagnosis of attention deficit hyperactivity disorder by using mr imaging and radiomics: a potential tool for clinicians. Radiology 2018;287: 631–2.

78. van Beek EJR, Kuhl C, Anzai Y, et al. Value of MRI in medicine: More than just another test? J Magn Reson Imaging 2019;49(7):e14–25.

Magnetic Resonance Spectroscopy for Psychiatry: Progress in the Last Decade

John D. Port, MD, PhD

KEYWORDS

- Psychiatry • Psychiatric disorder • Psychoradiology • Brain • Magnetic resonance spectroscopy
- Meta-analysis • Review

KEY POINTS

- Psychiatric disorders are quite common and can be quite severe; there is a critical clinical need to identify biomarkers of psychiatric disorders.
- Magnetic resonance spectroscopy (MRS) as a tool has identified potentially useful biomarkers of psychiatric illness but has limitations.
- Over the past decade, there have been significant advances in the way that psychiatric disorders are understood, classified, and researched as well as improvements in magnetic resonance imaging/MRS technology.
- A sufficient literature using MRS to study psychiatric disorders is now available, and several meta-analyses of that literature have found definite biochemical abnormalities in the brains of psychiatric patients.
- Although understanding of the underlying biochemistry of psychiatric disorders has improved, MRS as a tool has not yet proved helpful to individual patients with psychiatric symptoms.

INTRODUCTION

Psychiatric disorders are quite common in the population, with symptoms that can be loosely defined as disturbances in thought, emotions and/or behavior. The World Health Organization (WHO) began a systematic study of diseases including psychiatric disease in 1990 and since then has been tracking changes in disease prevalence in several more recent studies. The trends for various psychiatric diseases have been encouraging over the past 10 years. For example, death due to known mental and substance use disorders dropped 12.6% from a rate of 5.1:100,000 in 2005 to 4.5:100,000 in 2015. Significant progress was noted in the decrease in death rates of people with schizophrenia and alcohol use disorder, which each decreased 29.2% from 2005 to 2015. Deaths from drug use disorders increased 11.5%, largely due to the opioid epidemic. Although the rate of deaths due to self-harm (suicide due to all causes, including known mental illness) has decreased 16.3% from 13.7:100,000 in 2005 to 11.5:100,000 in 2015, the total number of deaths has remained stable across that time period, with approximately 1.2 million deaths/y (estimated at 2.15% of all deaths in 2015). Overall, in 2015, suicide was the fourteenth leading cause of death worldwide, surpassing deaths due to diabetes, liver cancer, breast cancer, and many other common diseases.[1]

With the progress made in decreasing the death rates from psychiatric illness, people with these illnesses are living longer, meaning that they have to suffer with and manage their symptoms for a longer period of time. In order to

Disclosure Statement: The author has nothing to disclose.
Department of Radiology, Mayo Clinic, 200 First Street Southwest, Rochester, MN 55905, USA
E-mail address: port.john@mayo.edu

neuroimaging.theclinics.com

quantify this suffering, the WHO has defined and measures years lived with disability, that is, years of life lived in less than optimal health. In 2015, the affective disorders (major depressive disorder [MDD] and bipolar disorder [BPD]) ranked third as the leading cause of years lived with disability, and anxiety disorders ranked ninth. In 2015, approximately 216 million people worldwide had received the diagnosis MDD and were trying to manage their often disabling symptoms.[2]

Despite great strides in diagnosing and treating most diseases over the last century, psychiatric "disorder" remains problematic. There are few objective measurable markers of psychiatric illness. Psychiatric "disorders" are syndromic, with psychiatric disorders defined in the *Diagnostic and Statistical Manual of Mental Disorders* (Fifth Edition) (*DSM-5*)[3] by a constellation of qualitative symptoms rather than by objective physiologic biomarkers. The lack of objective biomarkers for such disorders has created significant frustration for patients and clinicians alike and contributes to the demoralizing stigma of psychiatric illness.

Psychoradiology is an emerging discipline that applies the radiological techniques to psychiatric illnesses, an area in which Gong and colleagues have been its pioneers, and Gong is the "father of psychoradiology".[4,5] As one of the most important tools for psychoradiology, magnetic resonance spectroscopy (MRS) has long held great promise for the diagnosis and management of psychiatric disorders, because it is able to measure metabolic abnormalities in the brain thought to cause psychiatric symptoms. And, although significant progress has been made discovering metabolic markers of psychiatric illness, currently there is no MRS scan reliable enough to be used on an individual, clinical basis. This is not due to a lack of effort. A quick PubMed literature search looking for MRS and MDD (MR spectroscopy AND major depression AND brain) found approximately 135 articles from 1994 to 2008, and approximately 235 articles in the last decade from 2009 to 2019. Such research has occurred for other the psychiatric disorders as well, creating a wealth of MRS information.

A systematic review of these studies is no longer practical for a journal article. For a detailed review of the older studies prior to 2009, please consult Port and Puri.[6] This article focuses on the substantial developments in the field of psychiatric MRS in the past 10 years, presents select meta-analyses highlighting promising MRS findings, and closes with predictions about the future of psychiatric MRS.

A DECADE OF ADVANCES IN THE FIELD OF PSYCHIATRIC MAGNETIC RESONANCE SPECTROSCOPY
Updated Diagnostic Criteria

The diagnostic criteria for the various psychiatric disorders are defined in the *Diagnostic and Statistical Manual of Mental Disorders* (*DSM*), originally published in 1952. Over the years, various updates have been published in order to refine and clarify the different disorders. Although this has benefitted the accuracy and reproducibility of psychiatric diagnoses, these changes complicate comparisons of past and present literature, because it cannot be certain that studies of a given psychiatric disorder defined using different *DSM*s truly represent the same group of patients.

The most recent update occurred in 2013 when the American Psychiatric Association published the *DSM-V*.[3] This edition made major changes to the diagnostic criteria described in the previous *DSM* (Fourth Edition [IV]) (*DSM-IV*).[7] For example, the new criteria eliminate the subtypes of schizophrenia (paranoid, disorganized, catatonic, undifferentiated, and residual subtypes), eliminate the subsets of autism spectrum disorder (Asperger syndrome, classis autism, Rett syndrome, childhood disintegrative disorder, and pervasive developmental disorder not otherwise specified [NOS]) and combine alcohol abuse and alcohol dependence into a single alcohol use disorder. It can quickly be seen how it becomes difficult to compare studies with the experimental cohorts defined using the different versions of the *DSM*.

Furthermore, although this new edition had significant clinical and research implications, it also dramatically altered the way that people thought about mental health research. Thomas R. Insel (Director of the National Institute of Mental Health [NIMH] at the time) questioned the validity of the *DSM-V* classification scheme because "… diagnoses are based on a consensus about clusters of clinical symptoms …" as opposed to "… collecting the genetic, imaging, physiologic, and cognitive data to see how all the data – not just the symptoms – cluster and how these clusters relate to treatment response."[8] He declared at that time that the NIMH would no longer fund research projects that relied exclusively on *DSM-V* diagnostic criteria due to its lack of validity.

Updated Approach to Psychiatric Research

In 2010, several years before the *DSM-V* was released, Dr Insel proposed an alternative research methodology for psychiatric disorders called the Research Domain Criteria (RDoC).[9]

The idea is that psychiatric research should be structured into 5 major cognitive domains (negative valence systems, positive valence systems, cognitive systems, social processes, and arousal and regulatory systems), with research into a given domain performed by quantitatively evaluating 1 or more relevant units of analysis (genes, molecules, cells, circuits, physiology, behavior, and self-report). Over the next few years, teams of psychiatric scientists would work to define and refine the various psychiatric research domains, and the NIMH focused their funding efforts to grants which used the RDoC framework.

The articles generated from these first few grants are now published, and the question arises as to whether the research described in those articles is any better than the previous research performed using the *DSM-IV*, Text Revision, diagnostic criteria. Carcone and Ruocco[10] recently published a systematic review of 48 studies performed using the RDoC framework and ultimately concluded that it is too soon to tell if the framework made any significant impact on the way that psychiatric illness is studied. Regardless, comparing current to previous MRS studies has now become even more difficult.

Better Understanding of the Underlying Biology

The complex cellular biology of neurotransmission has been well studied over the past 50 years, but surprisingly it has been only recently that the relevant aspects of neurotransmission have been applied to MRS. It is well known that the most abundant excitatory neutotransmitter in the brain is glutamate, and the most abundant inhibitory neutotransmitter is γ-aminobutyric acid (GABA). Less well appreciated has been the cell-specific biochemistry of neurotransmitter synthesis. For example, as reviewed by Bak and colleagues,[11] neurons are incapable of synthesizing glutamate or GABA from glucose due to the lack of the enzyme pyruvate carboxylase. Instead, within neurons there is a more complex homeostasis involving the use of alternative substrates (eg, lactate and pyruvate) in the tricarboxylic acid cycle for de novo glutamate synthesis.

Furthermore, because synthesizing glutamate is metabolically expensive, recycling of glutamate once it has entered the synaptic cleft is preferred because it is much more energetically efficient. The glutamate/GABA-glutamine cycle has been proposed as the primary mechanism of neurotransmitter recycling in the brain (**Fig. 1**). Although this model for neurotransmitter recycling is generally well accepted, less well appreciated is the intrinsic intercellular transfer of ammonia produced in neurons when they convert glutamine to glutamate. Because neurons have no urea cycle, ammonia homeostasis between astrocytes and neurons is critical for neurotransmitter recycling and ammonia excretion from neurons. Much work remains to be done on neuron-astrocyte ammonia exchange and how glutamate/GABA-glutamine cycling has an impact on the symptoms in various psychiatric disorders.

MRS measures all of a given metabolite within the MRS voxel, regardless of its location. As such, it is impossible to use MRS to measure the amount of glutamate or GABA in a synaptic vessicle or a synaptic cleft. MRS studies of neurotransmitters over the past 20 years have perhaps naïvely assumed that glutamate levels correspond to neuronal activity, that is, the more glutamate is present within a given brain region, the greater the neuronal activity (specifically action potentials) in that region. Brain tissue contains high levels of glutamate, approximately 5 mmol/kg to 15 mmol/kg. Most of this glutamate is found in neurons, with the cytoplasmic glutamate levels reaching approximately 5 mM to 10 mM. Glutamate in the cytoplasm is thought to be primarily involved in cellular metabolism and energetics, specifically in the TCA cycle and mitochondria. It is now known that glutamate levels in the axon terminals are approximately 2 times to 3 times that of the cell bodies or dendrites,[12] probably due to the high level of mitochondria in the terminals. It is currently impossible, however, to determine—for an individual neuron—the fraction of total glutamate within the cytoplasm versus within the synaptic vesicles (glutamate available for neurotransmission) and the rate of release of vesicular glutamate into the synaptic cleft (glutamate actively involved in neurotransmission). Proton MRS, as it currently exists, will probably never be able to distinguish between these various compartments, and, therefore, the relative roles of glutamate in metabolism versus neurotransmission probably cannot be determined using proton MRS. Despite this limitation, the MRS literature in psychiatric illness has found significant differences in total glutamate in patients with psychiatric disorders; thus, although what is being affected cannot exactly be explained, glutamate homeostasis is definitely disrupted by those disorders.

Advances in Magnetic Resonance Spectroscopy Technology

Over the past decade, there have been substantial developments in MRS capabilities as a result of

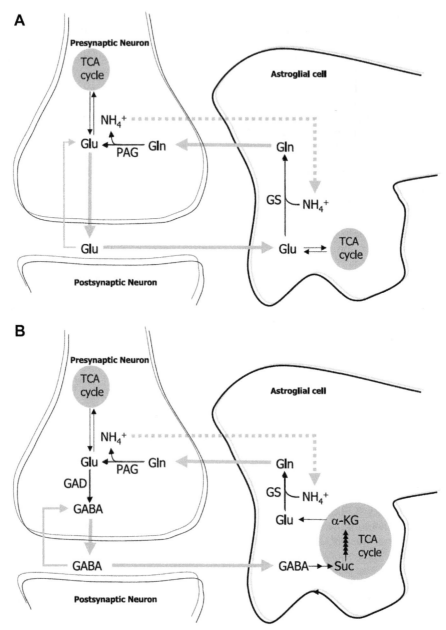

Fig. 1. Schematic representations showing the glutamate-glutamine cycle in a glutamatergic synapse (*A*) and a GABAergic synapse (*B*). In both synapses, the glutamate or GABA neurotransmitter is rapidly removed from the synaptic cleft by astrocytes and aminated to form glutamine. Glutamine is then transported back into the neuron where glutamate or GABA is regenerated for reuse in synaptic vesicles. aKG, alpha-ketoglutarate; GABA, gamma-amino butyric acid; GAD, glutamic acid decarboxylase; Gln, glutamine; Glu, glutamate; GS, glutamine synthase; PAG, phosphate-activated glutaminase; Suc, succinate; TCA, tricarboxylic acid cycle (*From* Bak LK, Schousboe A, Waagepetersen HS. The glutamate/GABA-glutamine cycle: aspects of transport, neurotransmitter homeostasis and ammonia transfer. J Neurochemistry 98:641-653, 2006, with permission.)

new technological advances in magnetic resonance (MR) hardware and software. Most of the early psychiatric spectroscopy work was performed on 1.5T magnetic resonance imaging (MRI) scanners using either stimulated echo acquisition mode (STEAM) or point-resolved spectroscopy (PRESS).[13,14] Although widely available and easy to use, these sequences suffer from several limitations,[15] including low signal-to-noise ratio (the primary reason STEAM is not used in brain MRS) and chemical shift offset arti-facts (significant differences in the measured locations of metabolites due to differences in the resonant frequencies of those metabolites). In parallel, it became clear that the most abundant metabolites (choline, creatine, and N-acetylaspartate [NAA]) were fairly stable in psychiatric illness, driving the field to focus on the neurotransmitters glutamate and GABA. Unfortunately, at 1.5T field strength, it is nearly impossible to separate glutamate from glutamine, limiting the value of the technique.

A MRI scanner technology progressed, the field shifted to using 3T MRI scanners, with better signal-to-noise ratio and larger spectral separation allowing for more accurate measurements of the metabolites. At 3T it became easy to separate glutamate from glutamine. The concept of optimizing an MRS sequence specifically for the measurement of glutamate became popular, leading to increasing heterogeneity in psychiatric MRS studies as researchers used different parameters in their MRS sequences.[16] Resolving GABA remained difficult, requiring innovative special sequences like Meshcher-Garwood point resolved spectroscopy (MEGA-PRESS)[17], which allows for the measurement of GABA but with additional limitations.[18]

In the past decade, 7T MRI scanners have become increasingly available, although widespread use in research studies has been limited due to the high cost of the scanners. At 7T, there is sufficient spectral separation to be able to resolve GABA without any complicated manipulations (Fig. 2), potentially leading to new and better literature on GABA abnormalities in psychiatric illness. Furthermore, although new sequences like semi-LASER have been developed to reduce chemical shift offset artifacts, 7T MRS suffers from many technical limitations that remain to be addressed.[19] In summary, there have been significant improvements in MRS technology over the past 30 years, and these improvements have made reliable measurements of glutamate and GABA possible. The challenge becomes comparing findings from earlier studies with current ones given the extremely heterogeneous scanner and sequence technology; in the end, many of the studies may need to be repeated using modern methods in order to make sense of their results.

Standardization of Magnetic Resonance Spectroscopy Quantification Methodology

Although MRI scanner and MRS sequence technology has become more heterogeneous over

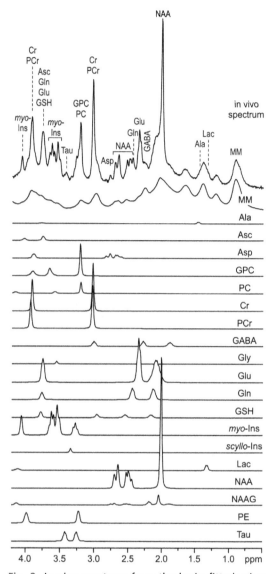

Fig. 2. In vivo spectrum from the brain fitted using LCModel. The top trace shows the raw spectrum; the GABA peak is easily identified just to the right of the glutamate (Glu) peak without the use of any special MRS sequence or postprocessing methodology. Ala, alanine; Asc, ascorbate; Asp, aspartate; Cr, creatine; GABA, gamma-amino butyric acid; Gln, glutamine; Glu, glutamate; Gly, glycine; GPC, glycerophophphorylcholine; GSH, glutathione; Lac, lactate; myo-Ins, myo-inositol; NAA, N-acetylaspartate; NAAG, N-acetylaspartylglutamate; PC, phosphorylcholine; PCr, phosphocreatine; Scyllo-Ins, scyllo-inositol; PE, phosphorylethanolamine; Tau, taurine. (From Godlewska BR, Clare S, Cowen PJ and Emir UE. Ultra-high-field magnetic resonance spectroscopy in psychiatry. Frontiers in Psychiatry 8:123, 2017, with permission.)

time, the analysis of MRS data have become fairly standardized. One major practice in the field has slowly fallen out of favor, specifically, that of using metabolite ratios rather than cerebrospinal fluid (CSF)-corrected metabolite concentrations. Although CSF does contain neurometabolites (glutamate, GABA, and lactate), in general these are present in micromolar concentrations. As such, CSF can be considered to contain no detectable metabolites with MRS, and any CSF that is included in the voxel artifactually reduces the measured brain metabolite values in that voxel. To deal with this issue, much of the early psychiatric MRS research was performed using the ratio of a given metabolite to creatine. As brain creatine levels were assumed to be constant in health and illness, any CSF in the voxel could simply be normalized out by dividing by the creatine concentration. Over the past decade, numerous studies have shown that the assumption of stable brain creatine is wrong, and absolute quantification by CSF correction of brain metabolites has become standard in the field.[20] This technique is now fairly easy to perform using free software, such as Freesurfer and FSL.[21]

Quantification of spectra has also become more standardized over time due to the wide availability of good automated versus semiautomated spectroscopy analysis software. The spectra in earlier psychiatric studies were quantified using simple peak integration, often with software developed in house by the authors.[22] As such, reproducing the results of prior studies was difficult at best due to the disparate data processing techniques. Over the past decade or so, most laboratories have switched to reliable spectral fitting software packages that use prior knowledge of metabolite peak structures to estimate metabolite concentrations. LCModel, jMRUI, and TARQUIN are the most commonly used software packages, and all give reliable, reproducible estimates of metabolite concentrations. Most modern psychiatric spectroscopy studies use one of these packages for data analysis.

SELECTED REVIEW OF PSYCHIATRIC MAGNETIC RESONANCE SPECTROSCOPY META-ANALYSES

Given the veritable explosion of psychiatric MRS research in the past 10 years, there is now enough material available to perform systematic meta-analyses of MRS data. A meta-analysis is a formal, quantitative unbiased study design used to systematically assess previous research studies in order to derive conclusions about a body of research. By statistically combining the results of those studies in a rigorous fashion, more precise estimates of brain abnormalities can become apparent, and better conclusions can be drawn from the results. The technique has many limitations, especially when combining multiple studies with data acquired from heterogeneous patient pools using heterogeneous MRS techniques (sequences and analysis methods). When performed well, however, meta-analysis is a powerful tool to detect and confirm metabolic abnormalities.

Schizophrenia

Schizophrenia is the most debilitating psychiatric illness. Unfortunately, a significant number of people with schizophrenia cannot cope with their disease and commit suicide. A positive aspect resulting from these tragic deaths is that because of the availability of brain tissue from these people, much is known about the biology of schizophrenia.

One of the models of psychotic symptoms in schizophrenia suggests that such symptoms result from imbalances in glutamate-GABA homeostasis, specifically, imbalances causes by dysfunction of the N-methyl-D-aspartate receptor (NMDAR) leading to excess glutamate release. As such, many investigators have evaluated glutamate dysfunction in various brain regions in patients with schizophrenia, unfortunately with mixed results. A recent meta-analysis by Merritt and colleagues[23] combined results from 59 different MRS studies, including data from 1686 patients and 1451 healthy controls. They found significant elevations of glutamate in the basal ganglia and thalamus, and significant elevations of glutamate plus glutamine (glx) in the basal ganglia and medial temporal lobe. Furthermore, they found elevated medial frontal glx levels in individuals at high risk for developing schizophrenia but not in those with first-episode psychosis or chronic schizophrenia. Conversely, they found elevated glx in the medial temporal lobe in people with chronic schizophrenia but not in those in the high-risk or first-episode groups. These regional differences support the ideas that schizophrenia is associated with excess glutamate neurotransmission, and that these glutamate abnormalities change over time as the disease progresses.

Postmortem studies of brain from people with schizophrenia consistently show decreased levels of neuronal mRNA for the GABA-synthesizing enzyme GAD67,[24] implying lower GABA levels in the brain during life. Several models of schizophrenia incorporate dysfunctional GABA signaling as a cause of some of the symptoms seen in the disease. Egerton and colleagues[25] recently performed a meta-analysis of 16 proton MRS studies of 526 patients and 538 controls. Their analysis failed to show any differences in GABA levels between healthy controls and patients with schizophrenia. A broader meta-analysis by Schür and colleagues[26] found similar results. Although these negative findings may seem to conflict with the extensive postmortem literature, it must be kept in mind that the data used in these 2 meta-analyses were acquired using suboptimal sequences (eg, MEGA-PRESS) on suboptimal MRI scanners (field strength <7T). As such, the lack of a positive result may simply reflect the limitations of the MRS techniques rather than the truth. Care must be taken when interpreting the results of meta-analyses because the nuances of MRS limitations often are lost in the discussion section of such articles.

More recently appreciated in the study of schizophrenia is the temporal progression of the disease. Specifically, often a patient suffers prodromal symptoms, abnormal thoughts/behaviors, and attenuated psychotic symptoms that do not reach criteria for schizophrenia at the time. Many of these patients go on to suffer an episode of psychosis, receiving the diagnosis of first-episode schizophrenia (FES); then, over time they progress to chronic schizophrenia. A substantial number of proton MRS studies have been performed on these prodromal subjects or subjects with high-risk of developing schizophrenia based on family history. Brugger and colleagues[27] performed a meta-analysis evaluating MRS findings separated by stage of illness. They found significant reductions in NAA in the frontal lobes, temporal lobes, and thalami regardless of disease stage in the schizophrenic groups relative to healthy controls. Furthermore, in high-risk individuals, NAA levels were lower in the thalami. This thalamic NAA finding was replicated in a separate meta-analysis by Iwata and colleagues,[28] further supporting the idea of a thalamic neuronal abnormality in schizophrenia.

Mood Disorders

Mood disorders, specifically MDD and BPD refer to a group of illnesses characterized by the elevation or lowering of a person's mood in a way that is inconsistent with the person's circumstances. Typically, mood disorders interfere with normal everyday life, and these disturbances can last for weeks or months at a time. The glutamate hypothesis of depression was proposed in the 1990s, theorizing that glutamate levels are decreased in depression, perhaps due to reduced neurotransmission and/or NMDAR function because depressive symptoms cleared

with NMDAR agonists. With proper treatment, glutamate levels were proposed to increase, normalizing to levels found in healthy controls. A recent meta-analysis by Moriguchi and colleagues[29] evaluated glutamate levels in people with MDD. A review of 49 studies of 1180 patients and 1066 healthy controls found significantly decreased glx in the medial prefrontal cortex of patients relative to controls, supporting the glutamate hypothesis of depression.

In contrast, glutamate levels are thought to be elevated in patients with BPD which is a syndrome involving both episodes of depression and mania. A meta-analysis by Gigante and colleagues[30] looked at 17 studies of patients with BPD. They found increased glx levels in the frontal lobes (as well as all brain regions evaluated) of bipolar patients relative to healthy controls, regardless of medication status, thus supporting that hypothesis. Furthermore, 2 meta-analyses by Chitty and colleagues[31] found additional evidence of elevated glutamate levels in the frontal lobes of bipolar patients with impaired mismatch negativity, a neurophysiological measurement used as an index of NMDAR function. Together these studies provide mounting evidence supporting an abnormal frontal lobe glutamate system.

One of the challenges of using MRS to study mood disorders is the concept of trait versus state. Specifically, it has become challenging to determine disease trait—a chronic, reproducible diagnosis, such as MDD or BPD, that can be measured regardless of the mood of the patient—versus disease state—a relatively acute, fluctuating mood condition, such as mania or depression. Clinically speaking, it is fairly easy to determine the current mood state of the patient, but determining the disease trait remains a difficult and critical problem, because proper treatment of a given disorder relies on properly diagnosing the disorder. As an example, both MDD and BPD type 2 suffer recurrent episodes of depression; in the absence of a history of mania, the disorders are in many ways indistinguishable, making appropriate treatment difficult at best. Davis and colleagues[32] have proposed a classification system of biomarkers of neuropsychiatric disease in order to tease out these effects, but past research, including the studies included in these recent meta-analyses, has not rigorously controlled for trait and state, making interpretation of the results difficult.

SUMMARY

Over the past decade, there have been significant advances in both MRS technology and the quality of psychiatric MRS studies. Furthermore, the number of psychiatric MRS studies is now sufficient such that high-quality meta-analyses can be performed. These meta-analyses have provided solid statistical evidence of metabolite abnormalities in various brain regions for the different psychiatric disorders, helping to refine understanding of the causes of these disorders. This is good news indeed; the stigma of psychiatric disease is starting to fade as the concrete scientific evidence of brain abnormality in psychiatric illness continues to grow.

Unfortunately, although scientific understanding of these disorders has advanced, MRS as a technique has not yet proved helpful to individual patients with psychiatric illness. There are many reasons for the lack of adequate MRS biomarkers. First, although the reliability and reproducibility of the MRI scanners, MRS sequences, and analysis techniques has significantly improved over the past decade, there remains significant variability in the measurement of neurotransmitters (glutamate and GABA) and their metabolic products (glutamine). Much like psychiatric MRS studies shifted from 1.5T to 3T scanners, over the next few years there will likely be a shift to 7T MRI scanners, hopefully improving reproducibility. Next, psychiatric MRS research needs to better control for numerous patient factors: state versus trait of a given presumed disease and disease stage (prodromal vs early vs chronic) at the time of the scan remain significant confounders for the analysis of the MRS results. The RDoC framework provides a potentially better way to organize such research, although many investigators argue that the *DSM-V* diagnostic criteria are just as valid as the RDoC domains. Finally, as understanding of the underlying biology continues to improve, innovative MRS techniques, such as functional MRS, nonproton (^{31}phosphorus or ^{13}carbon) MRS, and provocative testing (eg, ketamine infusion while performing MRS), may identify new biologically relevant biomarkers.

Ironically, one of the motivations for studying brain chemistry using MRS was a failure of traditional anatomic imaging to find any significant differences between normal and disease. For example, several anatomic MRI studies using MR volumetry failed to find any significant differences in ventricle size between mood disorder patients and healthy controls. As a modality, anatomic MRI scans have failed to yield any actionable biomarkers for psychiatric illness. Although MRS has had more success in identifying abnormalities than anatomic imaging, perhaps as Gong and

colleagues and Biswal and colleagues suggest in their articles in this issue, the future of psychiatric imaging may shift to the functional MRI realm. As functional MRI techniques improve, extracting functional networks and seeing how they change over time will improve. It will be curious to see what the next decade of MRI/MRS research discovers in the quest to find clinically useful biomarkers of psychiatric illness.

REFERENCES

1. Global, regional, and national life expectancy, all-cause mortality, and cause-specific mortality for 249 causes of death, 1980-2015: a systematic analysis for the Global Burden of Disease Study 2015. Lancet 2016;388:1459–544.
2. Global, regional, and national incidence, prevalence, and years lived with disability for 310 diseases and injuries, 1990-2015: a systematic analysis for the Global Burden of Disease Study 2015. Lancet 2016;388:1545–602.
3. American Psychiatric Association. Diagnostic and statistical manual of mental disorders (fifth edition). Arlington (VA): American Psychiatric Publishing; 2013.
4. Gong Q, Lui S, Sweeney JA. A selective review of cerebral abnormalities in patients with first-episode schizophrenia before and after treatment. Am J Psychiatry 2016;173:232–43.
5. Huang X, Gong Q, Sweeney JA, et al. Progress in psychoradiology, the clinical application of psychiatric neuroimaging. Br J Radiol 2019;92:20181000.
6. Port J, Puri B. Magnetic resonance spectroscopy in psychiatry. In: Gillard JH, Waldman AD, Barker PB, editors. Clinical MR Neuroimaging: Physiological and Functional Techniques. Cambridge: Cambridge University Press; 2009. p. 566–92.
7. American Psychiatric Association. Diagnostic and statistical manual of mental disorders (fourth edition, text revision). Washington, DC: American Psychiatric Publishing; 2000.
8. Insel T. Transforming diagnosis. Director's blog. Rockville (MD): National Institute of Mental Health; 2013.
9. Insel T, Cuthbert B, Garvey M, et al. Research domain criteria (RDoC): toward a new classification framework for research on mental disorders. Am J Psychiatry 2010;167:748–51.
10. Carcone D, Ruocco AC. Six years of research on the national institute of mental health's research domain criteria (RDoC) initiative: a systematic review. Front Cell Neurosci 2017;11:46.
11. Bak LK, Schousboe A, Waagepetersen HS. The glutamate/GABA-glutamine cycle: aspects of

transport, neurotransmitter homeostasis and ammonia transfer. J Neurochem 2006;98:641–53.

12. Featherstone DE. Intercellular glutamate signaling in the nervous system and beyond. ACS Chem Neurosci 2010;1:4–12.

13. Frahm J, Merboldt K-D, Hänicke W. Localized proton spectroscopy using stimulated echoes. J Magn Reson 1987;72:502–8.

14. Bottomley PA. Spatial localization in NMR spectroscopy in vivo. Ann N Y Acad Sci 1987;508:333–48.

15. Moonen CT, von Kienlin M, van Zijl PC, et al. Comparison of single-shot localization methods (STEAM and PRESS) for in vivo proton NMR spectroscopy. NMR Biomed 1989;2:201–8.

16. Hancu I. Optimized glutamate detection at 3T. J Magn Reson Imaging 2009;30:1155–62.

17. Mescher M, Tannus A, Johnson M, et al. Solvent suppression using selective echo dephasing. J Magn Reson 1996;123:226–9.

18. Mullins PG, McGonigle DJ, O'Gorman RL, et al. Current practice in the use of MEGA-PRESS spectroscopy for the detection of GABA. Neuroimage 2014;86:43–52.

19. Henning A. Proton and multinuclear magnetic resonance spectroscopy in the human brain at ultrahigh field strength: a review. Neuroimage 2018; 168:181–98.

20. Jansen JF, Backes WH, Nicolay K, et al. 1H MR spectroscopy of the brain: absolute quantification of metabolites. Radiology 2006;240:318–32.

21. Quadrelli S, Mountford C, Ramadan S. Hitchhiker's guide to voxel segmentation for partial volume correction of in vivo magnetic resonance spectroscopy. Magn Reson Insights 2016;1–9. https://doi.org/10.4137/MRI.S32903.

22. Mierisova S, Ala-Korpela M. MR spectroscopy quantitation: a review of frequency domain methods. NMR Biomed 2001;14:247–59.

23. Merritt K, Egerton A, Kempton MJ, et al. Nature of glutamate alterations in schizophrenia: a meta-analysis of proton magnetic resonance spectroscopy studies. JAMA Psychiatry 2016;73:665–74.

24. Glausier JR, Lewis DA. GABA and schizophrenia: Where we stand and where we need to go. Schizophr Res 2017;181:2–3.

25. Egerton A, Modinos G, Ferrera D, et al. Neuroimaging studies of GABA in schizophrenia: a systematic review with meta-analysis. Transl Psychiatry 2017; 7:e1147.

26. Schür RR, Draisma LW, Wijnen JP, et al. Brain GABA levels across psychiatric disorders: a systematic literature review and meta-analysis of (1) H-MRS studies. Hum Brain Mapp 2016;37:3337–52.

27. Brugger S, Davis JM, Leucht S, et al. Proton magnetic resonance spectroscopy and illness stage in schizophrenia–a systematic review and meta-analysis. Biol Psychiatry 2011;69:495–503.

28. Iwata Y, Nakajima S, Plitman E, et al. Neurometabolite levels in antipsychotic-naive/free patients with schizophrenia: a systematic review and meta-analysis of 1H-MRS studies. Prog Neuropsychopharmacol Biol Psychiatry 2018;86: 340–52.

29. Moriguchi S, Takamiya A, Noda Y, et al. Glutamatergic neurometabolite levels in major depressive disorder: a systematic review and meta-analysis of proton magnetic resonance spectroscopy studies. Mol Psychiatry 2019;24:952–64.

30. Gigante AD, Bond DJ, Lafer B, et al. Brain glutamate levels measured by magnetic resonance spectroscopy in patients with bipolar disorder: a meta-analysis. Bipolar Disord 2012;14:478–87.

31. Chitty KM, Lagopoulos J, Lee RS, et al. A systematic review and meta-analysis of proton magnetic resonance spectroscopy and mismatch negativity in bipolar disorder. Eur Neuropsychopharmacol 2013; 23:1348–63.

32. Davis J, Maes M, Andreazza A, et al. Towards a classification of biomarkers of neuropsychiatric disease: from encompass to compass. Mol Psychiatry 2015;20:152–3.

Imaging-Based Subtyping for Psychiatric Syndromes

Elena I. Ivleva, MD, PhD[a],*, Halide B. Turkozer, MD[a], John A. Sweeney, PhD[b]

KEYWORDS

- Psychiatric disorders • Neuroimaging • Psychoradiology • MR imaging • Disease subtypes
- Biomarkers

KEY POINTS

- Major psychiatric syndromes as currently defined are highly heterogeneous and show considerable overlap in clinical features, disease course, neurobiological markers, genetic susceptibility and treatment response.
- Identifying disease subtypes based on psychoradiology, within and across psychiatric syndromes, offers novel perspectives potentially relevant to development of more precise diagnostic algorithms and targeted treatments.
- Considerable challenges exist in incorporating research imaging approaches into clinical practice of psychiatry.
- Multidisciplinary efforts are needed to bridge the gap between research and clinical practice and to demonstrate translational applicability of imaging-based subtyping approaches in psychiatry.

INTRODUCTION

In contrast to other areas of medicine, considerable gaps exist between neuroimaging research and clinical practice in psychiatry. Extensive research demonstrates significant alterations captured with multimodal brain imaging in various psychiatric conditions. Along with cognitive and electrophysiological approaches, neuroimaging methods have been central to the neurobiological conceptualization of psychiatric disorders. In fact, imaging research was central to shifts from psychological to biological models of serious mental illness in the 1970s and 1980s.[1] Imaging tools provide advantages over other methods in light of their wide availability and ability to provide noninvasive quantitative data on structural, functional, and chemical alterations in the brain. Moreover, imaging approaches have demonstrated considerable potential for capturing biologically homogeneous subgroups of patients with complex brain disorders, offering pathways for novel translational and clinical applications.[2–4]

Nevertheless, despite considerable advances in neuroimaging research, brain imaging is still not a widely used tool in diagnostic algorithms for psychiatric disorders. Multiple hindrances contribute to this persisting research-clinical practice gap, including but not limited to the innate complexity of psychiatric disorders, overwhelming clinical and biological heterogeneity of the current diagnostic constructs, poor diagnostic specificity, and lack of established reliability of imaging findings from large-scale validation studies, as well as considerable practical demands related to

Disclosure Statement: All authors declare no related conflict of interest.
Funded by: NIH/NIMH. Grant Number(s): MH077851; MH103368.
[a] Department of Psychiatry, UT Southwestern Medical Center, 5323 Harry Hines Boulevard, NC5, Dallas, TX 75390, USA; [b] Department of Psychiatry, University of Cincinnati, 2600 Clifton Avenue, Cincinnati, OH 45221, USA
* Corresponding author. Department of Psychiatry, UT Southwestern Medical Center, 5323 Harry Hines Boulevard, NE5.110H, Dallas, TX 75390-9127.
E-mail address: elena.ivleva@utsouthwestern.edu

implementation of quantitative neuroimaging tools in clinical practice. The developing field of psychoradiology, pioneered by Gong and his colleagues (https://radiopaedia.org/articles/psychoradiology),[2,5,6] undertakes the challenging task of incorporating radiological approaches into the daily workflow of psychiatry.

With enhanced knowledge of molecular and structural determinants of medical conditions, diagnostic classifications in most fields of medicine have been largely transformed from nosology/symptom-based to biologically based taxonomies. Yet, diagnostic formulations in psychiatry remain at a far less advanced level. Instead of grouping patients by combined laboratory and clinical evidence into well-validated disease entities that warrant specific treatments, psychiatric diagnoses broadly characterize patients into clinically overlapping and biologically heterogeneous conditions.[7] The marked heterogeneity within and across psychiatric syndromes also manifests as discordance between emerging biomarker-informed disease constructs and conventional symptom-based diagnoses.[8–10] This limitation hinders progress in elucidating disease mechanisms, developing biologically informed methods to predict outcomes, and exploiting novel approaches to advance precision medicine. Most importantly, the lack of biologically informed disease definitions has been a bottleneck in the development of mechanistic therapeutic targets.[11,12]

Because biological heterogeneity within psychiatric syndromes is large, brain alterations are similar across diagnoses, and biological mechanisms of illness so poorly understood, the role for diagnostic radiology in relation to psychiatry is complex in relatively novel ways. First, there are no obvious imaging targets suitable for direct clinical translation. Although neuroimaging research has identified a wide range of abnormalities in different psychiatric disorders, they often involve relatively modest and widely distributed alterations across the brain that have poor diagnostic specificity. Second, alterations associated with psychiatric disorders are rarely seen on visual inspection, and require fairly complex quantitative analysis of parameters like regional volume and cortical thickness, none of which are immediately available in clinical practice. Third, syndromal diagnoses need to be parsed into biologically discrete entities as in other fields of medicine. This latter point implies that radiological approaches need to be applied collaboratively with psychiatric researchers in a research context to define biologically homogeneous subgroups of patients within syndromes and to evaluate the utility of imaging data for predicting prognosis and

differential treatment response.[11,13] However, this is possible based on the psychoradiological theory of Gong and colleagues, in which brain structural alteration leads to clinical syndromes via impact on widely distributed functional connectivity.[2,5,14–16]

Efforts to develop clinically useful imaging markers for complex psychiatric syndromes such as schizophrenia, bipolar disorder, and attention-deficit/hyperactivity disorder (ADHD), have generally failed, largely because of substantial biological heterogeneity of these syndromes.[8,17] Success of psychoradiology is more likely to be achieved by demonstrating a unique ability to capture biologically homogenous and specific "disease units" (and corresponding subgroups of patients) based on brain alterations detectable with imaging, despite phenomenological similarities across the subgroups, similar to other medical conditions, for example, diabetes type 1 versus 2. Making progress in these directions requires a multidisciplinary effort and a considerable shift in conceptual framework in both psychiatric and radiology research and clinical practice.

In this article, we discuss imaging approaches designed to capture neurobiologically distinct disease constructs across major psychiatric syndromes. We present a conceptual review of the most robust and important findings from studies that use imaging data as subtyping measures for defining distinct disease subtypes, as well as external validators of subtypes derived from other neurobiological measures. We specifically focus on approaches that have a high relevance to psychiatric disease manifestations, functional outcomes, and treatment planning. We emphasize cross-diagnostic and dimensional approaches. Furthermore, we discuss current challenges in translating psychiatric imaging into clinical practice and strategies to move forward in the evolution of psychoradiology that will benefit from combined efforts of psychiatry and radiology investigators and clinicians.

SUBTYPING OF PSYCHIATRIC SYNDROMES BASED ON BRAIN IMAGING BIOMARKERS

Various imaging approaches, including structural MR imaging, diffusion tensor imaging (DTI), functional MR imaging (fMR imaging), and MR spectroscopy (MRS), have been used to study psychiatric patients. An extensive neuroimaging literature demonstrates considerable heterogeneity of imaging findings *within,* and overlaps *between,* psychiatric syndromes (eg, McTeague and colleagues[18]). Therefore, transdiagnostic studies are of great importance, as they provide strategies to capture more biologically-homogenous disease units irrespective of or "masked" by current clinical diagnoses.[8,19]

One neuroimaging approach is to parse biological heterogeneity based on imaging features (eg, functional connectivity, fractional anisotropy), and then characterize emerging subgroups with respect to relevant symptoms and clinical outcomes.[4] Hermens and colleagues[20] used DTI-based fractional anisotropy (FA) to derive imaging-based subgroups across a broad range of psychiatric diagnoses, including psychotic, affective (depressive, bipolar) and anxiety disorders. They demonstrated 3 clusters characterized by specific alterations in FA values. Notably, these clusters did not correspond to clinical diagnoses, and showed similar cognitive and behavioral/symptom abnormalities.

A more sophisticated approach, capturing both biological and behavioural manifestations of psychopathology, is to link specific brain alterations to phenomenological manifestations across multiple diagnostic categories in order to identify patient groups with distinct "bio-behavioral" profiles. Stefanik and colleagues[21] derived such "bio-behavioral" constructs integrating cortical thickness, subcortical volume, and DTI-based tractography data with cognitive and clinical characteristics across individuals with schizophrenia spectrum disorders, autism spectrum disorders, bipolar disorder, and healthy individuals. They identified 4 novel groups with distinct "neural circuit-cognitive" profiles, and validated these constructs using independent imaging and functional measures. The "circuit-cognitive" constructs demonstrated greater differentiation on structural circuit nodes and social functioning than traditional diagnostic classes. Goodkind and colleagues[22] identified a shared pattern of gray matter loss in the anterior insula and dorsal anterior cingulate across 6 diverse diagnostic groups including schizophrenia, bipolar disorder, depression, addiction, obsessive-compulsive disorder, and anxiety. Furthermore, they demonstrated that the regions involved in this "transdiagnostic structural abnormality pattern" formed an interconnected network during task-based and resting state fMR imaging, and showed associations with poor cognitive functioning.[22]

Ivleva and colleagues[23] identified broad and overlapping patterns of gray matter volume reductions across the "psychosis dimension" in probands with schizophrenia, schizoaffective and psychotic bipolar disorder. Similar gray matter changes were found in biological relatives of patient probands with mild psychosis manifestations. Lifetime duration of psychosis and psychotic symptom severity inversely correlated with gray matter volumes in several neocortical (eg, frontal, temporal, insular) and subcortical (thalamus, basal ganglia) regions,[23] suggesting a potential value of MR data for estimating clinical prognosis. Targeting functional brain networks, Xia and colleagues[10] identified correlated patterns of functional connectivity and symptom dimensions in a large sample of youth. Using sparse canonical correlation analysis, they revealed 4 dimensions, "mood," "psychosis," "fear," and "externalizing behavior," which were associated with distinct patterns of functional connectivity.

A recent meta-analysis of task-based fMR imaging studies tracking brain activity during a broad array of sensory, motor and cognitive tasks-applied in patients with diverse diagnoses revealed a shared transdiagnostic pattern of regional activation abnormalities localized to prefrontal cortex, anterior insula, intraparietal sulcus, and midcingulate/presupplementary motor area.[18] These regions correspond to the "multiple-demand network" that is critically important for adaptive, flexible cognition.

Dimensionally-focused imaging studies have demonstrated broader overlap spanning not only various disease cohorts but also healthy populations.[9,24,25] Price and colleagues[9] used a fMR imaging-based connectivity approach to parse functional connectivity profiles across depressed and healthy adults during "positive mood induction" (ie, exposure to emotionally positive stimuli). They identified 2 functional connectivity-based groups exhibiting hypoconnectivity or hyperconnectivity, which spanned the "depression-healthy" dimension. The subgroup characterized by hyperconnectivity demonstrated higher self-reported depressive symptoms and lower sustained positive mood during the induction. Costa Dias and colleagues[24] demonstrated distinct subgroups among typically developing children and children with ADHD based on functional connectivity characteristics within the reward network. Gates and colleagues[25] identified 5 subgroups based on functional connectivity networks in a dimensionally organized sample of ADHD and typically developing children. Two of these subgroups were composed of mainly ADHD cases; however, approximately a third of children with ADHD were spread across 3 other subgroups, which predominantly contained typically developing children.

Transdiagnostic and dimensional studies are few; nevertheless, neurobiologically informed disease constructs that have been generated by these studies share critically important characteristics and teach useful lessons. First, the findings consistently demonstrate that the imaging-based subgroups do not map well onto traditional symptom-based diagnoses. This has important implications for the unlikely success of simple "MR profiles for existing disorders" approaches, which represents most of the relevant literature. Second, some imaging-based constructs appear to capture groups of cases with extremes of neural features.[9,25] These subgroups may represent "tipping points" that mark a transition to either a more severe or qualitatively different pathology.[7] Identification of such points and examining their relationship with risk and resilience factors are of potential clinical importance.[7] Third, dimensional approaches have demonstrated neurobiological overlaps beyond the disease realm, extending to healthy populations. Identifying mechanisms that allow "healthy" individuals to compensate for a biological feature indicative of disease risk may inform paths to individualized treatments and disease prevention.

IMAGING APPROACHES AS INDEPENDENT VALIDATORS OF DISEASE SUBTYPES DERIVED FROM OTHER NEUROBIOLOGICAL MEASURES

Technological advances in clinical neuroscience provide powerful methods (eg, electrophysiological, neuroimaging) to characterize the neurobiological diversity of psychiatric disorders. However, development of optimal strategies for combining largely variable findings from methodologically diverse studies to inform clinically translatable knowledge has been challenging. Using these methods for disease subtyping and subsequently validating and extending subtype constructs with neuroimaging methods offers advantages for clinical translation purposes. In this section, we review studies that use *neuroimaging techniques as independent validators* to capture the biological distinctiveness of experimental disease constructs derived from other biomarker-based tools.

To our knowledge, Sun and colleagues[3] were the first to subtype psychiatric disorders based on imaging features using an unsupervised machine-learning technique/algorithm, and they identified 2 distinct subtypes of schizophrenia using DTI. This is a milestone from the perspective of imaging-based subtyping, as they are the first to parse psychiatric disorder subtypes based on neuroimaging and machine-learning approaches. Subsequently Drysdale and colleagues[26] defined depression subtypes in individual patients via a similar approach.

Another leading effort that incorporated this strategy, along with broader psychosis biomarker-focused goals, was implemented by the Bipolar-Schizophrenia Network for Intermediate Phenotypes (B-SNIP) consortium.[27] The B-SNIP has undertaken a novel strategy of applying a dense biomarker battery to a large, dimensionally acquired psychosis sample to (1) characterize biological heterogeneity underlying psychotic syndromes, and (2) identify subgroups of psychosis cases based on their distinctive neurobiological profiles irrespective of clinical diagnosis. In a sample of psychosis probands (including schizophrenia, schizoaffective, and psychotic bipolar I disorders, n = 711), their first-degree relatives (n = 883), and healthy subjects (n = 278), Clementz and colleagues[8] performed a series of multivariate taxometric analyses using a broad battery of cognitive, eye movement, and electroencephalogram (EEG)-based biomarkers, and identified 3 neurobiologically distinct groups, the "B-SNIP Biotypes" (for details on biotype development see Clementz and colleagues[8]). Biotype1 cases were characterized by significantly impaired cognitive function and sensorimotor reactivity; Biotype2 cases had reduced cognitive function but exaggerated sensorimotor reactivity, primarily evident in increased intrinsic EEG activity; and Biotype3 cases showed normal cognitive function and only modestly diminished sensorimotor reactivity, compared with healthy controls. Similar, albeit attenuated, neurobiological profiles were observed in relatives consistent with patient biotype classification; this suggests familial and/ or heritable characteristics of the Biotypes. Furthermore, conventional diagnoses did not correspond to the Biotypes: all 3 targeted diagnoses were represented in all biotype groups, only with a slight predominance of schizophrenia cases in Biotype1 and bipolar cases in Biotype3.[8]

Using a whole-brain voxel-wise gray matter density approach, Ivleva and colleagues[28] demonstrated extensive and diffuse gray matter reductions (predominant in frontal, temporal, and cingulate cortex) in Biotype1. Biotype2 showed intermediate and more localized reductions, with the largest effects in insula and fronto-temporal regions, whereas Biotype3 showed small, highly localized reductions, mainly in anterior limbic regions. Biological relatives grouped by their respective probands' biotype demonstrated distinctive regional effects: broadly distributed gray matter reductions in relatives of Biotype1, with the strongest effects in anterior (fronto-temporal, cingulate) regions; predominantly posterior (visual and auditory sensory cortices, cerebellum) reductions in Biotype2 relatives; and normal gray matter structure in Biotype3 relatives. Biotypes showed stronger group separation based on gray matter density characteristics, and were a stronger predictor of gray matter density change, compared with conventional diagnoses.[28]

Meda and colleagues[29] used resting state fMR imaging to identify impaired functional connectivity in the Biotypes in 9 functional networks linked to diverse cognitive functions, for example, cognitive control, working memory, attention, and introspective thought maintenance. All biotype groups showed reduced connectivity across the networks, except for one: the cuneus-occipital network showed reductions in connectivity in biotypes1 and 2, but not biotype3. In addition, biotype1 and biotype2 relatives showed reduced connectivity in the fronto-parietal network, compared with controls. Biotypes performed marginally better in discriminating psychosis subgroups compared with conventional diagnoses, based on resting state functional connectivity deficits.[29]

Mothi and colleagues[30] investigated the utility of machine-learning approaches for delineating psychosis subgroups in the B-SNIP sample. Integrating both clinical and biomarker-based data (EEG, cognition), they used an unsupervised learning algorithm and identified 3 distinct clusters. They used brain structure, eye movement, and social functioning data as independent validators for the observed subgroups. The greatest cortical thinning was depicted in group 1; group 2 showed milder impairments; whereas little to no significant differences were observed for group 3, compared with controls. The 3 conventional psychosis syndrome diagnoses were represented in all novel subgroups, again highlighting the non-specificity of imaging findings across conventional diagnoses.[30]

A complementary approach is to initially parse disease heterogeneity based on clinical features alone (eg, symptom clusters, lifetime history, disease course), and investigate their biological correlates using neuroimaging approaches. Maglanoc and colleagues[31] studied a large sample of individuals with and without lifetime history of depression, and identified 5 subgroups with distinct depression and anxiety symptom profiles, which cut across diagnostic boundaries. Similar to the B-SNIP psychosis biotype constructs, participants with or without history of depression were represented in all novel subgroups. Furthermore, these subgroups demonstrated distinct resting state functional connectivity patterns, specifically in the fronto-temporal network. These findings suggest that data-driven clustering methods, even based on dimensionally organized symptom data alone, may capture more biologically relevant disease constructs than conventional diagnoses.[31]

Dimensional approaches offer unique advantages in capturing the profound clinical and biological heterogeneity evident not only in disease populations but also in healthy individuals.[32] Van Dam and colleagues[32] identified data-driven phenotypes based on behavioral features that represent different functional domains personality/temperament, symptom features, interpersonal functioning, and behavioral tendencies—in a community-ascertained sample. Using a hybrid hierarchical clustering method, they identified a nested hierarchy of homogenous participant groups. The algorithm identified 2 groups based on functional adaptiveness: adaptive versus maladaptive. Moreover, the 2 groups demonstrated differences in functional connectivity in several networks, including limbic, thalamic, basal ganglia, and somatomotor regions.[32]

Taken together, growing evidence indicates the substantial biological heterogeneity associated with current diagnostic formulations of psychiatric syndromes, and advanced biomarker and computational tools could perform the imaging-based subtyping for psychiatric syndromes. These strategies may help link different levels of brain system pathology and elucidate within-level and between-level relationships across clinical manifestations, biomarkers, and molecular disease markers. Neuroimaging tools, which provide rich structural and functional information through noninvasive approaches, are essential to these efforts, both as a means of disease subtyping and external validators to develop novel, biologically informed disease formulations.

IMAGING-BASED SUBTYPING RELEVANT TO PROGNOSIS AND TREATMENT OUTCOMES

Most available treatments in psychiatry were discovered coincidentally and are not targeting identified disease mechanisms. Treatment approaches informed by objective, measurable brain-based biomarkers are currently lacking.

"Precision medicine" is an emerging concept that aims to incorporate an individual patient's symptom, biological, and environmental factors into clinical decision making.[33,34] Although precision medicine approaches have become routine in other fields (eg, infectious and cardiovascular diseases), they remain at an early stage of development in psychiatry. The ultimate goal of "precision psychiatry" is to identify neural signatures that can inform clinical prognosis and treatment response to particular interventions a priori, with a high level of exactness.[13,33] Implementation of the approach will depend on success in the challenging task of elucidating mechanisms of psychiatric disorders, or in the absence of full disease mechanisms, identification of outcome predictors or modifiable treatment targets. Similar to other complex disorders with largely unknown mechanisms (eg, cancer), substantial progress in clinical outcomes can be made via implementation of specific treatments targeting known aspects of the disorder, for example, herceptin in treatment of HER2 overexpressing breast cancer.

Growing evidence supports neuroimaging as one of the most promising approaches for precision psychiatry.[5,35,36] Several recent reviews[35,37–39] outline review progress in the implication of neuroimaging methods in predicting treatment response, transition to advanced disease stage, and predicting functional outcomes. Various neuroimaging methods have been used to identify patterns that predict treatment response, including structural and functional MR imaging, DTI, and MRS.[35] Studies have reported imaging biomarkers of therapeutic response in major depressive disorder (MDD), including structural and functional characteristics within the frontostriatal-limbic network.[38,40] A recent meta-analysis demonstrated that increased activity in the anterior cingulate cortex was predictive of a higher likelihood of improvement in response to pharmacologic and psychotherapy interventions in MDD.[40] Furthermore, 2 separate meta-analyses[40,41] identified reduced hippocampal volume as a predictor of poorer treatment response and lower remission rates in individuals with depression. In addition to predictors of pharmacologic treatment response,[41–44] neuroimaging studies have offered biomarkers of response to neuromodulation (eg, electroconvulsive therapy,[45,46] transcranial magnetic stimulation),[26,47–49] and psychotherapy[50] in MDD.

In bipolar disorder, most studies have focused on neuroimaging predictors of treatment response to lithium and other mood stabilizers. Several studies reported associations between increased hippocampal, amygdala, and cortical volumes/thickness and good lithium response in individuals with bipolar disorder (for a recent review see Porcu and colleagues).[51] Structural and functional alterations in emotion processing and broader brain networks have been linked to various mood stabilizer effects and/or treatment response,[51] including in pediatric bipolar samples.[4,52,53] Machine-learning approaches applied to multimodal imaging data have demonstrated high classification accuracies (more than 80%) for predicting lithium response in first-episode mania.[54] Similar approaches in schizophrenia indicated greater ventricular volumes,[55] diminished fronto-temporal gray matter volumes,[56] and reduced white matter integrity in various tracts[57,58] as neuroimaging correlates of poorer response to antipsychotic treatments (for a recent review, see Tarcijonas and Sarpal).[59] Although fewer in number, studies in other psychiatric disorders (eg, ADHD, posttraumatic stress disorder[60–62]) demonstrated the use of neuroimaging biomarkers as predictors of treatment response.

Another rapidly developing and promising area in "precision psychiatry" research is identification of potential neural markers that are predictive of future onset of psychosis in individuals at "clinically high risk" (CHR).[39] Regionally specific alterations in medial temporal lobe and prefrontal cortex volumes and white matter integrity have been associated with psychosis conversion (for a comprehensive review, see Gifford and colleagues[39]). Koutsouleris and colleagues[63] demonstrated that structural alterations in a broad set of neocortical regions and cerebellum were predictive of functional outcome in CHR individuals. Das and colleagues[64] reported that disorganized gyrification network properties predicted transition to psychosis in CHR individuals with higher than 80% accuracy. Cao and colleagues,[65] using fMR imaging data from the North American Prodrome Longitudinal Study, showed significantly increased connectivity in a cerebello-thalamo-cortical circuit in CHR individuals who later developed psychosis. Bossong and colleagues[66] used MRS to demonstrate that MRS-based hippocampal glutamate levels were significantly elevated in CHR individuals who subsequently converted to psychosis or had poor functional outcome at follow-up. These studies offer potential strategies towards the identification of specific neural signatures that may inform clinical decision making in "at risk" individuals with the aim of identifying individuals for intervention to prevent the onset of psychosis.

Considerable limitations, however, warrant caution in interpretation of these early efforts. The substantial clinical and biological heterogeneity of available disease constructs, for example, MDD or schizophrenia, limit diagnostic specificity of imaging findings. Likewise, other target groups (eg, CHR samples) are characterized by substantial variability in biological features, disease course, and functional outcomes.[39,67] Most studies to date are based on small to modest sample sizes, which may lead to overoptimistic predictor estimates.[35,68] Alternative strategies built on identification of biologically homogeneous groups in large, transdiagnostic, multimodal datasets, and subsequent investigation of their predictive potential are needed to use neural and clinical heterogeneity to increase the accuracy and replicability of precision medicine in psychiatry.

SUMMARY AND FUTURE DIRECTIONS

Parsing disease subtypes based on neuroimaging approaches, within and across complex psychiatric syndromes, can provide more precise diagnostic algorithms and targeted treatments. Progress in research can move the field past early "proof of concept" studies. However, challenges will need to be addressed including advances in psychiatric nosology relying more on brain-based features, developing clinically useful and valid biomarkers, and practical limitations. Substantial work is needed to bridge the gap between research and clinical practice to demonstrate the translational applicability of imaging findings in psychiatry. This work is needed to address crucial questions:

- Are imaging-based disease subtypes reproducible in independent research and clinical samples? Do they provide specific targets suitable for clinical translation?
- Do subtypes derived from different imaging modalities correspond to each other? If not, can the information be combined for clinical decision making?
- Do subtype constructs derived in patients at different disease stages (eg, early vs chronic course) correspond to each other? How do psychiatric treatments impact imaging findings?
- Could subtypes derived via sophisticated (and costly) imaging tools be detected by less costly biomarkers?

To begin to tackle these challenges, there is a critical need for replication studies that incorporate multimodal biomarkers. Large-scale biomarker-focused consortia have made progress, but more studies along these lines are needed.[27,69,70] Future efforts are needed to parse biological heterogeneity of psychiatric syndromes to guide successful clinical translation. In addition, longitudinal studies are needed to investigate the prognostic value of imaging features. To date, pharmacologic target and clinical trial studies incorporating radiology tools are few, and are typically limited by small samples and single imaging modalities (eg, fMR imaging or DTI). Furthermore, much more basic work is necessary in linking human in vivo biomarkers (eg, those captured with imaging) to potential molecular targets via animal models or live cell studies. Cumulatively, these strategies may move the field closer to elucidating disease mechanisms and exploiting mechanistically informed therapeutic targets: the bases for successful clinical translation.

Another challenge is the limited current application of available imaging tools in routine practice of psychiatry. In contrast to many other fields of medicine in which radiology tools are the cornerstone of diagnostic algorithms, imaging data are rarely used to support psychiatric diagnoses except to exclude neurologic disease. Experimental research biomarker batteries (eg, the B-SNIP) are complex and costly, and require substantial technical and analytical expertise, and there is a great need for further development in automatic quantification tools for rapid analysis of imaging data. Such tools may be useful not only for clinical practice but also for the pharmacologic industry to stratify patients for trials and establish target engagement.

Ultimately, to successfully address the challenging task of establishing clinical utility, the field of psychoradiology will have to move beyond group-level analysis and bring imaging markers to an individual patient level. This calls for sophisticated computational approaches, which would allow biomarker characterization and "biotyping" in individual patients, in real time, with subsequent application of these biomarkers as a means to guide clinical decision making. Changes in radiology and psychiatric training, and in insurance reimbursement policies, will be needed to support objective brain measures as part of routine clinical workup and are examples of challenging tasks lying ahead.

To conclude, significant challenges remain for direct clinical translation of neuroimaging research in psychiatry, though none are insurmountable in light of fast progress in other fields of medicine towards similar translational goals. The developing field of psychoradiology offers unique paths to tackle these challenges via multidisciplinary efforts that bridge research and clinical practice.[6] If successful, these efforts may generate stronger diagnostic algorithms and offer novel therapeutic targets for psychiatric disorders.

REFERENCES

1. Cunningham Owens DG, Johnstone EC, Bydder GM, et al. Unsuspected organic disease in chronic schizophrenia demonstrated by computed tomography. J Neurol Neurosurg Psychiatry 1980;43(12):1065–9.
2. Lui S, Zhou XJ, Sweeney JA, et al. Psychoradiology: the frontier of neuroimaging in psychiatry. Radiology 2016;281(2):357–72.

3. Sun H, Lui S, Yao L, et al. Two patterns of white matter abnormalities in medication-naive patients with first-episode schizophrenia revealed by diffusion tensor imaging and cluster analysis. JAMA Psychiatry 2015;72(7):678–86.

4. Zhang W, Xiao Y, Sun H, et al. Discrete patterns of cortical thickness in youth with bipolar disorder differentially predict treatment response to quetiapine but not lithium. Neuropsychopharmacology 2018;43(11):2256–63.

5. Gong Q. Response to Sarpal et al.: importance of neuroimaging biomarkers for treatment development and clinical practice. Am J Psychiatry 2016; 173(7):733–4.

6. Huang X, Gong Q, Sweeney JA, et al. Progress in psychoradiology, the clinical application of psychiatric neuroimaging. Br J Radiol 2019;92(1101): 20181000.

7. Cuthbert BN, Insel TR. Toward the future of psychiatric diagnosis: the seven pillars of RDoC. BMC Med 2013;11:126.

8. Clementz BA, Sweeney JA, Hamm JP, et al. Identification of distinct psychosis biotypes using brain-based biomarkers. Am J Psychiatry 2016;173(4): 373–84.

9. Price RB, Lane S, Gates K, et al. Parsing heterogeneity in the brain connectivity of depressed and healthy adults during positive mood. Biol Psychiatry 2017;81(4):347–57.

10. Xia CH, Ma Z, Ciric R, et al. Linked dimensions of psychopathology and connectivity in functional brain networks. Nat Commun 2018;9(1):3003.

11. Keshavan MS, Lawler AN, Nasrallah HA, et al. New drug developments in psychosis: challenges, opportunities and strategies. Prog Neurobiol 2017; 152:3–20.

12. Linden D. Biological psychiatry: time for new paradigms. Br J Psychiatry 2013;202(3):166–7.

13. Insel TR, Cuthbert BN. Medicine. Brain disorders? Precisely. Science 2015;348(6234):499–500.

14. Gong Q, Lui S, Sweeney JA. A selective review of cerebral abnormalities in patients with first-episode schizophrenia before and after treatment. Am J Psychiatry 2016;173(3):232–43.

15. Lui S, Deng W, Huang X, et al. Association of cerebral deficits with clinical symptoms in antipsychotic-naive first-episode schizophrenia: an optimized voxel-based morphometry and resting state functional connectivity study. Am J Psychiatry 2009;166(2):196–205.

16. Tregellas J. Connecting brain structure and function in schizophrenia. Am J Psychiatry 2009;166(2): 134–6.

17. Sun H, Chen Y, Huang Q, et al. Psychoradiologic utility of MR imaging for diagnosis of attention deficit hyperactivity disorder: a radiomics analysis. Radiology 2018;287(2):620–30.

18. McTeague LM, Huemer J, Carreon DM, et al. Identification of common neural circuit disruptions in cognitive control across psychiatric disorders. Am J Psychiatry 2017;174(7):676–85.

19. Tamminga CA, Pearlson GD, Stan AD, et al. Strategies for advancing disease definition using biomarkers and genetics: the bipolar and schizophrenia network for intermediate phenotypes. Biol Psychiatry Cogn Neurosci Neuroimaging 2017; 2(1):20–7.

20. Hermens DF, Hatton SN, White D, et al. A data-driven transdiagnostic analysis of white matter integrity in young adults with major psychiatric disorders. Prog Neuropsychopharmacol Biol Psychiatry 2019; 89:73–83.

21. Stefanik L, Erdman L, Ameis SH, et al. Brain-behavior participant similarity networks among youth and emerging adults with schizophrenia spectrum, autism spectrum, or bipolar disorder and matched controls. Neuropsychopharmacology 2018;43(5):1180–8.

22. Goodkind M, Eickhoff SB, Oathes DJ, et al. Identification of a common neurobiological substrate for mental illness. JAMA Psychiatry 2015;72(4):305–15.

23. Ivleva EI, Bidesi AS, Keshavan MS, et al. Gray matter volume as an intermediate phenotype for psychosis: Bipolar-Schizophrenia Network on Intermediate Phenotypes (B-SNIP). Am J Psychiatry 2013;170(11):1285–96.

24. Costa Dias TG, Iyer SP, Carpenter SD, et al. Characterizing heterogeneity in children with and without ADHD based on reward system connectivity. Dev Cogn Neurosci 2015;11:155–74.

25. Gates KM, Molenaar PC, Iyer SP, et al. Organizing heterogeneous samples using community detection of GIMME-derived resting state functional networks. PLoS One 2014;9(3):e91322.

26. Drysdale AT, Grosenick L, Downar J, et al. Resting-state connectivity biomarkers define neurophysiological subtypes of depression. Nat Med 2017; 23(1):28–38.

27. Tamminga CA, Ivleva EI, Keshavan MS, et al. Clinical phenotypes of psychosis in the bipolar-schizophrenia network on intermediate phenotypes (B-SNIP). Am J Psychiatry 2013;170(11): 1263–74.

28. Ivleva EI, Clementz BA, Dutcher AM, et al. Brain structure biomarkers in the psychosis biotypes: findings from the bipolar-schizophrenia network for intermediate phenotypes. Biol Psychiatry 2017;82(1): 26–39.

29. Meda SA, Clementz BA, Sweeney JA, et al. Examining functional resting-state connectivity in psychosis and its subgroups in the bipolar-schizophrenia network on intermediate phenotypes cohort. Biol Psychiatry Cogn Neurosci Neuroimaging 2016; 1(6):488–97.

30. Mothi SS, Sudarshan M, Tandon N, et al. Machine learning improved classification of psychoses using clinical and biological stratification: update from the bipolar-schizophrenia network for intermediate phenotypes (B-SNIP). Schizophr Res 2018. [Epub ahead of print].

31. Maglanoc LA, Landro NI, Jonassen R, et al. Data-driven clustering reveals a link between symptoms and functional brain connectivity in depression. Biol Psychiatry Cogn Neurosci Neuroimaging 2019; 4(1):16–26.

32. Van Dam NT, O'Connor D, Marcelle ET, et al. Data-driven phenotypic categorization for neurobiological analyses: beyond DSM-5 labels. Biol Psychiatry 2017;81(6):484–94.

33. Fernandes BS, Williams LM, Steiner J, et al. The new field of 'precision psychiatry'. BMC Med 2017; 15(1):80.

34. National Research Council. Toward precision medicine: building a knowledge network for biomedical research and a new taxonomy of disease. Washington (DC): National Academies Press; 2011.

35. Janssen RJ, Mourao-Miranda J, Schnack HG. Making individual prognoses in psychiatry using neuroimaging and machine learning. Biol Psychiatry Cogn Neurosci Neuroimaging 2018;3(9):798–808.

36. Sarpal DK, Lencz T, Malhotra AK. In support of neuroimaging biomarkers of treatment response in first-episode schizophrenia. Am J Psychiatry 2016; 173(7):732–3.

37. Dazzan P, Arango C, Fleischacker W, et al. Magnetic resonance imaging and the prediction of outcome in first-episode schizophrenia: a review of current evidence and directions for future research. Schizophr Bull 2015;41(3):574–83.

38. Fonseka TM, MacQueen GM, Kennedy SH. Neuroimaging biomarkers as predictors of treatment outcome in major depressive disorder. J Affect Disord 2018;233:21–35.

39. Gifford G, Crossley N, Fusar-Poli P, et al. Using neuroimaging to help predict the onset of psychosis. Neuroimage 2017;145(Pt B):209–17.

40. Fu CH, Steiner H, Costafreda SG. Predictive neural biomarkers of clinical response in depression: a meta-analysis of functional and structural neuroimaging studies of pharmacological and psychological therapies. Neurobiol Dis 2013;52:75–83.

41. Colle R, Dupong I, Colliot O, et al. Smaller hippocampal volumes predict lower antidepressant response/remission rates in depressed patients: a meta-analysis. World J Biol Psychiatry 2018;19(5): 360–7.

42. Gyurak A, Patenaude B, Korgaonkar MS, et al. Frontoparietal activation during response inhibition predicts remission to antidepressants in patients with major depression. Biol Psychiatry 2016;79(4): 274–81.

43. Kraus C, Klobl M, Tik M, et al. The pulvinar nucleus and antidepressant treatment: dynamic modeling of antidepressant response and remission with ultra-high field functional MRI. Mol Psychiatry 2019; 24(5):746–56.

44. Liu J, Xu X, Luo Q, et al. Brain grey matter volume alterations associated with antidepressant response in major depressive disorder. Sci Rep 2017;7(1): 10464.

45. Levy A, Taib S, Arbus C, et al. Neuroimaging biomarkers at baseline predict electroconvulsive therapy overall clinical response in depression: a systematic review. J ECT 2019;35(2):77–83.

46. Redlich R, Opel N, Grotegerd D, et al. Prediction of individual response to electroconvulsive therapy via machine learning on structural magnetic resonance imaging data. JAMA Psychiatry 2016; 73(6):557–64.

47. Avissar M, Powell F, Ilieva I, et al. Functional connectivity of the left DLPFC to striatum predicts treatment response of depression to TMS. Brain Stimul 2017; 10(5):919–25.

48. Fan J, Tso IF, Maixner DF, et al. Segregation of salience network predicts treatment response of depression to repetitive transcranial magnetic stimulation. Neuroimage Clin 2019;22:101719.

49. Weigand A, Horn A, Caballero R, et al. Prospective validation that subgenual connectivity predicts antidepressant efficacy of transcranial magnetic stimulation sites. Biol Psychiatry 2018;84(1):28–37.

50. Marwood L, Wise T, Perkins AM, et al. Meta-analyses of the neural mechanisms and predictors of response to psychotherapy in depression and anxiety. Neurosci Biobehav Rev 2018;95:61–72.

51. Porcu M, Balestrieri A, Siotto P, et al. Clinical neuroimaging markers of response to treatment in mood disorders. Neurosci Lett 2018;669:43–54.

52. Kafantaris V, Spritzer L, Doshi V, et al. Changes in white matter microstructure predict lithium response in adolescents with bipolar disorder. Bipolar Disord 2017;19(7):587–94.

53. Wegbreit E, Ellis JA, Nandam A, et al. Amygdala functional connectivity predicts pharmacotherapy outcome in pediatric bipolar disorder. Brain Connect 2011;1(5):411–22.

54. Fleck DE, Ernest N, Adler CM, et al. Prediction of lithium response in first-episode mania using the LIThium Intelligent Agent (LITHIA): pilot data and proof-of-concept. Bipolar Disord 2017;19(4):259–72.

55. Lieberman J, Chakos M, Wu H, et al. Longitudinal study of brain morphology in first episode schizophrenia. Biol Psychiatry 2001;49(6):487–99.

56. Quarantelli M, Palladino O, Prinster A, et al. Patients with poor response to antipsychotics have a more severe pattern of frontal atrophy: a voxel-based morphometry study of treatment resistance in schizophrenia. Biomed Res Int 2014;2014:325052.

57. Samanaite R, Gillespie A, Sendt KV, et al. Biological predictors of clozapine response: a systematic review. Front Psychiatry 2018;9:327.
58. Zeng B, Ardekani BA, Tang Y, et al. Abnormal white matter microstructure in drug-naive first episode schizophrenia patients before and after eight weeks of antipsychotic treatment. Schizophr Res 2016; 172(1–3):1–8.
59. Tarcijonas G, Sarpal DK. Neuroimaging markers of antipsychotic treatment response in schizophrenia: an overview of magnetic resonance imaging studies. Neurobiol Dis 2018;131:104209.
60. Kim JW, Sharma V, Ryan ND. Predicting methylphenidate response in ADHD using machine learning approaches. Int J Neuropsychopharmacol 2015; 18(11):pyv052.
61. Szeszko PR, Yehuda R. Magnetic resonance imaging predictors of psychotherapy treatment response in post-traumatic stress disorder: a role for the salience network. Psychiatry Res 2019;277:52–7.
62. Yang YJD, Allen T, Abdullahi SM, et al. Brain responses to biological motion predict treatment outcome in young adults with autism receiving Virtual Reality Social Cognition Training: Preliminary findings. Behav Res Ther 2017;93:55–66.
63. Koutsouleris N, Kambeitz-Ilankovic L, Ruhrmann S, et al. Prediction models of functional outcomes for individuals in the clinical high-risk state for psychosis or with recent-onset depression: a multimodal, multisite machine learning analysis. JAMA Psychiatry 2018;75(11):1156–72.
64. Das T, Borgwardt S, Hauke DJ, et al. Disorganized gyrification network properties during the transition to psychosis. JAMA Psychiatry 2018;75(6):613–22.
65. Cao B, Cho RY, Chen D, et al. Treatment response prediction and individualized identification of first-episode drug-naive schizophrenia using brain functional connectivity. Mol Psychiatry 2018. [Epub ahead of print].
66. Bossong MG, Antoniades M, Azis M, et al. Association of hippocampal glutamate levels with adverse outcomes in individuals at clinical high risk for psychosis. JAMA Psychiatry 2019;76(2):199–207.
67. Nelson B, Yuen HP, Wood SJ, et al. Long-term follow-up of a group at ultra high risk ("prodromal") for psychosis: the PACE 400 study. JAMA Psychiatry 2013;70(8):793–802.
68. Varoquaux G. Cross-validation failure: small sample sizes lead to large error bars. Neuroimage 2018; 180(Pt A):68–77.
69. Cannon TD, Chung Y, He G, et al, North American Prodrome Longitudinal Study Consortium. Progressive reduction in cortical thickness as psychosis develops: a multisite longitudinal neuroimaging study of youth at elevated clinical risk. Biol Psychiatry 2015;77(2):147–57.
70. van Erp TGM, Walton E, Hibar DP, et al. Cortical brain abnormalities in 4474 individuals with schizophrenia and 5098 control subjects via the enhancing neuro imaging genetics through meta analysis (ENIGMA) consortium. Biol Psychiatry 2018;84(9): 644–54.

Individual-Specific Analysis for Psychoradiology

Hesheng Liu, PhD[a],*, William J. Liu, BSc[b], Danhong Wang, MD, PhD[a],
Louisa Dahmani, PhD[a]

KEYWORDS

- Psychoradiology • MR imaging • Functional connectivity • Individual differences
- Personalized medicine

KEY POINTS

- The gold standard for study design and diagnostic guidelines no longer fits contemporary needs and restricts the ability of current investigators to meticulously investigate brain disorders in detail.
- Individual-specific functional neuroimaging analysis should address many of the concerns with the current methods of investigation and should be a core component of psychoradiology in the future.
- Individual-specific psychoradiology may facilitate biomarker discovery, enable brain-based patient stratification, and lead to personalized treatments.

INTRODUCTION

Advancements in numerous radiological modalities, such as functional magnetic resonance imaging (fMRI), have provided insight regarding the mechanisms of mental disorders. These neuroimaging methods have contributed to a robust body of literature concerning potential neural substrates of mental disorders, and in particular the development of psychoradiology as an emerging subspecialty of neuroradiology. These advances have begun to show potential to play a role in guiding diagnostic decisions and therapeutic planning in psychiatric patients.[1–3] This is an addition to the psychoradiological theory of Gong et al, in which brain structural alteration leads to clinical syndromes via impact on widely distributed functional connectivity.[4–7] However, the neural mechanisms for most psychiatric disorders remain obscure. At present, there is contention surrounding the ideal criteria for the clinical diagnosis of psychiatric disorders and whether the current guidelines are suitable for practical use.[8,9] Whether psychiatrists and researchers transition from a strictly categorical approach based on symptoms to one that also considers dimensions derived from neuroimaging data will have large implications for future clinical practice in psychiatry. This progression will require further developments in neuroimaging techniques to enable accurate characterization of the individual subjects' brains. This article addresses how individual-specific analysis can affect psychiatric research and how it may be used as a component of psychoradiology in the future.

WHY INDIVIDUAL-SPECIFIC ANALYSIS IS IMPORTANT

Recent advancements in technical and analytical brain imaging tools have allowed researchers to

Funding: NIH, grant numbers 1R01DC017991, 7R01NS091604, K01MH111802; NIHMS-ID, 1539818.
[a] Athinoula A. Martinos Center for Biomedical Imaging, Department of Radiology, Massachusetts General Hospital, Harvard Medical School, 149 13th Street, Suite 2301, Charlestown, MA 02129, USA; [b] Department of Neuroscience, Grossman Institute of Neurobiology, The College, University of Chicago, 5812 South Ellis Avenue, MC 0912, Suite P-400, Chicago, IL 60637, USA
* Corresponding author.
E-mail address: hesheng.liu@mgh.harvard.edu

investigate patients at the individual level, opening the door for personalized medicine and treatment. These investigations are fairly new in the field of psychiatry, in which studies designed to find group-level differences are the gold standard, whether that be case-control studies, cohort studies, or randomized control trials. These types of investigations are prevalent because they are often straightforward, and, in the early phase of psychiatric research, significant findings can potentially be generalized to large populations, after which individual variance in brain alterations can be exploited to guide clinical practice for individual patients. Nearly all neuropsychiatric imaging research has involved investigating group differences in brain characteristics between groups of patients and healthy control subjects. However, even before individual-specific neuroimaging analysis was feasible, many researchers emphasized the importance of personalized investigations,[10,11] and attempts to interpret results derived from individualized analysis have increased within the last few years. This increase is crucial for the translational shift from research to clinical practice that is central to the developing clinical field of psychoradiology.

Interest in investigating individual differences is justified. Every individual is unique, and this is exemplified by the considerable interindividual variability in neural activity and structural neuroanatomy in human brains. For instance, Braga and Buckner[12] investigated the functional network organization of 4 healthy individuals by scanning each subject 24 times. Simply investigating the commonalities between the subjects by evaluating the data as a group resulted in a loss of notable organizational characteristics that may have strong implications in a variety of psychiatric disorders. Braga and Buckner's[12] work raises concerns regarding the reliability and practicality of group-averaged data. In parallel, Fisher and colleagues' recent work[13] argues that future investigators should categorically analyze the ergodicity of the processes being studied by comparing the mean and variance of the interindividual and intraindividual distributions, citing the potential for cases of improper statistical inference. They contend that, similar to how a cross-sectional sample must be representative of a population before a generalizable claim can be made, the data derived from within an individual must also be representative of the individual's data over a time period before an inference can be established. Thus, findings from studies that have used aggregated data from single time point sampling may be less compelling than originally regarded and

investigators should be cautious about extrapolating findings observed at the group level to the individual.

Although individual variability provides incentives for the rapid development of individual-specific approaches, individual-level functional brain imaging was previously deemed impractical because of several validity and reliability concerns.[14] For example, task-based fMR imaging is known to suffer from poor signal/noise ratio (SNR), limited test-retest reliability,[15–17] and inconsistency with respect to invasive electrical cortical stimulation, causing many investigators to question its clinical utility. A recent meta-analysis using task fMR imaging data from 1088 participants indicated a poor overall reliability (mean intraclass correlation coefficient = .397).[18] The investigators argued that "commonly used task-fMRI measures are not currently suitable for brain biomarker discovery or individual differences research in cognitive neuroscience." As a result, the field has been under scrutiny for having a replicability crisis, the observation that the findings of a large number of studies are often not corroborated by follow-up studies.

However, recent advancements in computational neuroimaging may provide approaches to address the concerns of individual-specific analysis delineated earlier. For instance, using resting-state fMR imaging, Wang and colleagues[19] showed that functional brain organization may be reliably mapped over time within individuals. Finn and colleagues[20] showed that individual functional connectivity can act as a fingerprint for each patient, suggesting that an important component of interindividual variability is robust, stable, and reproducible. Similarly, Tavor and colleagues[21] showed that it is possible to predict the task-induced brain activity of unseen individuals using a model that is based on individual variability in resting-state brain connectivity, further highlighting the intrinsic link between each individual's neural organization and function. Thus, individual-specific imaging analysis based on these computational approaches may be able to reliably capture an individual's brain characteristics at a given time point, which can be an exceptionally useful in psychoradiology.

CHARACTERIZING AN INDIVIDUAL SUBJECT'S BRAIN FOR BIOMARKER DISCOVERY

Characterizing individual subjects' brain organization is at the core of psychoradiology. Mueller and colleagues[22] performed a meta-analysis and showed that functional connections predicting individual differences in the behavioral and cognitive domains are predominantly located in the association cortex, including the language, executive control, and attention networks, which are known to be wired more differently between individuals than the unimodal regions. In psychiatric patients, symptoms are largely related to abnormal activity in cognitive networks that are substantially variable across individuals, thus the exploration of brain-behavior associations requires accurate mapping in each individual. Wang and colleagues[19] developed a brain network parcellation approach based on resting-state functional connectivity and showed its ability in localizing individuals' major functional networks. Subject-specific functional network organization was determined using an iterative adjusting algorithm, which was initially guided by a population-based atlas and an intersubject variability map preestimated in the population. Critically, the influence of the population-based atlas on the individual brain parcellation was not identical for every subject or every brain region, and was flexibly adjusted based on the known distribution of intersubject variability and the SNR distribution in a particular subject. Specifically, a weighting strategy was applied in which the population-based atlas had less impact than the individual subject's data on brain regions known to have high levels of intersubject variability, or brain regions showing a good SNR in a particular subject. The influence of the population-based information gradually decreases as the iteration proceeds, allowing the final map to be completely driven by the individual subject's data. This strategy successfully leverages the knowledge of organizational principles shared by the population and at the same time maximizes the use of information embedded in an individual subject's data. This approach greatly improved the within-subject reproducibility of the functional maps and was able to reveal the intersubject variability in network distribution. Within the same subject, the results showed an average reproducibility of 82.4% across sessions, as measured by the Dice coefficient. At the same time, the technology is sensitive to characteristics of the individual and reflects intersubject variability. Between any 2 individuals, the Dice coefficient was only 60.5%. Importantly, functional networks localized using this parcellation technology could be validated by invasive cortical stimulation mapping in a small group of surgical patients (n = 8).

Capitalizing this subject-specific functional network parcellation, Li and colleagues[23] recently proposed a method to reliably identify a set of discrete, homologous functional regions across individuals. This method allows investigators to dissociate individual variability in size, position, and connectivity of functional regions. They found that previously reported intersubject variability in functional connectivity maps was largely explained by variability in position of the functional regions, but was less related to the variability in connectivity strength among these regions. Moreover, the investigators found that individual differences in connectivity architecture can predict individual differences in task-evoked activations. As a result, the functional alignment based on these homologous regions can improve the statistical power of fMRI activation analyses across various tasks. Critically, they showed that not only the connectivity strength but also the size and position of these individually specified regions can capture the idiosyncrasies of individuals and are able to better predict individual differences in cognitive ability than conventional approaches based on brain templates. These results are echoing recent findings of Kong and colleagues,[24] who reported that topological features of brain networks are behaviorally relevant and may predict cognition, personality, and emotion.

The ability to map homologous functional regions across individuals will facilitate the exploration of brain-symptom relations. In a recent study, Wang and colleagues[25] localized 116 cortical regions of interest (ROIs) in 76 patients with schizophrenia or schizoaffective disorder (ie, primary nonaffective psychosis) to estimate positive symptom severity, as measured on positive subscore of the Positive and Negative Syndrome Scale (PANSS). The PANSS positive scores predicted by connectivity were significantly correlated with the PANSS positive scores observed in patients ($r = 0.50$, $P = .004$), whereas the same analysis using atlas-based ROIs was unable to predict the PANSS positive scores. Moreover, using the same participants and procedure, the investigators trained separate models to predict severity of negative symptoms (ie, PANSS negative subscores) and mania, using total scores on the Young Mania Rating Scale (YMRS). Functional connectivity among the individually specified ROIs was able to predict scores on PANSS negative ($r = 0.35$, $P = .033$) and YMRS ($r = 0.51$, $P = .011$). As was the case for positive symptom estimation, these models performed at or near chance when relying on atlas-defined ROIs. An important test of a model's specificity is how well it might be able to distinguish domains of dysfunction, as opposed to reflecting general mental disorder. In comparing the sets of connections that were most predictive of positive and negative symptoms, they were completely nonoverlapping.

These findings show that such an individualized approach provides information that is both individually predictive and specific to different domains of dysfunction in psychosis.

A core question arising from categorical and dimensional models of mental disorders is the extent to which neural circuit dysfunction seen in these conditions reflects (categorical) disease cause, (dimensional) symptom presentation, or some combination of the two. Previous work using atlas-based methods to extract connectivity estimates failed to identify any differences between network abnormalities in bipolar and primary psychotic patients.[26] Using the individualized methods described earlier, Wang and colleagues[25] trained models to predict PANSS positive scores in 55 patients with bipolar disorder. Although connectivity derived using this approach was still able to robustly predict positive symptom levels in the bipolar sample, the set of connections used to predict PANSS positive levels in this group was almost completely nonoverlapping with those identified for patients with primary nonaffective psychosis. Moreover, models using data combining the 2 patient subgroups failed to predict PANSS positive or negative ratings when the diagnostic label was not included as a feature in the model.

Using a similar data-driven, individual-level approach, Brennan and colleagues[27] attempted to predict global and dimension-specific symptoms of obsessive-compulsive disorder (OCD) based directly on functional connectivity. They constructed an individualized connectome for each of 41 patients with OCD receiving intensive residential treatment who had received fMRI scans. A support vector machine for a regression model was trained to predict global OCD symptom severity as measured by the Yale-Brown Obsessive Compulsive Scale (Y-BOCS), and scores on each of the 4 categories on the Dimensional Obsessive-Compulsive Scale (DOCS1–4: 1, concerns about germs and contamination; 2, concerns about being responsible for harm, injury, or bad luck; 3, unacceptable thoughts; 4, concerns about symmetry, completeness, and the need for things to be just right) based on ROI-to-ROI connectivity. Y-BOCS scores predicted by the individualized connectome correlated significantly with participants' actual Y-BOCS scores ($r = 0.528$, $P < .001$). Most importantly, they identified a set of connections that collectively predicted DOCS1 scores ($r = 0.333$; $P = .033$) and a separate set of connections that predicted DOCS2 scores ($r = 0.337$; $P = .031$). Notably, functional connectivity analyses using atlas-based ROIs failed to predict either DOCS1 or DOCS2.

Taken together, although these findings are subject to future replications in independent populations, this emerging research direction that focuses on individualized functional analysis has already shown great promise in revealing meaningful biomarkers for a variety of psychiatric symptoms.

INVESTIGATING INDIVIDUAL-SPECIFIC TREATMENTS

Current clinical methods to treat psychiatric disorders have room for improvement.[28] There is evidence that suggests suboptimal performance of contemporary treatments for mental illness may be rooted in individual differences. Individualized psychoradiology can facilitate the development of a personalized treatment strategies to improve clinical efficacy. A good example of individual variability in psychiatric patients is seen in treatment response to neuromodulation such as repetitive transcranial magnetic stimulation (rTMS). Although it offers promise as a viable treatment for depression and OCD,[29,30] several studies have found the standard application of rTMS to be suboptimal.[31–33] Fox and colleagues[34] observed that there is notable heterogeneity in patients with depression regarding their functional connectivity, and ideal rTMS targets may be best generated based on each individual's unique functional brain organization. In a more recent study on antidepressant rTMS treatment, Weigand and colleagues[35] examined functional connectivity between each patient's rTMS stimulation site in the dorsolateral prefrontal cortex and subgenual cingulate. Clinical efficacy was predicted by stimulation sites that were more negatively correlated with subgenual cingulate. Remarkably, these findings were replicated in an independent dataset. Although this study did not use the subjects' own fMRI data to quantify connectivity but used normative population data, it nevertheless emphasized the importance of individualized rTMS targeting. Taken together, these studies all suggest that individual-specific analysis can play a sizable role in improving the efficacy of contemporary psychiatric treatments, and individualized target approaches have potential that needs to be actively pursued.

CLASSIFICATION OF PSYCHIATRIC DISORDERS

Individualized analysis of functional imaging may lead to a more objective, and presumably more accurate, stratification of psychiatric patients. For instance, it provides potentially useful functional biomarkers for psychiatric subtyping. For the first time, Drysdale and colleagues[36] defined depression subtypes in individual patients, while Sun and colleagues[37] were the first to subtype patients with psychiatric disorders based on structural imaging features using an unsupervised machine learning technique/algorithm.[36,37]

Most researchers in psychiatry appreciate the complexity of severe mental illnesses and the need to go beyond the narrow definitions of the Diagnostic and Statistical Manual of Mental Illness (DSM) and the International Classification of Diseases (ICD). These definitions reflect a tradition based on clinical observations borne out of an era that largely predated significant knowledge about the brain. As a result, diagnosis based on these definitions often leads to a high level of heterogeneity within and across psychiatric disorders. For example, McTeague and Lang[38] observed that patients diagnosed with posttraumatic stress disorder can be separated into groups at polar opposites on the scale for reactivity, suggesting that the disease encompasses 2 distinct disorders with divergent biological mechanisms. A recent study showed that individuals diagnosed with depression can be subdivided into 4 biotypes by identifying intrinsic irregularities in limbic and frontostriatal functional connectivity networks in the brain.[36] Different groups responded differently to rTMS, suggesting that each biotype may have a different underlying disorder and requires individualized treatment. One approach to overcoming this historical barrier is the Research Domain Criteria (RDoC), part of the 2008 NIMH Strategic Plan to "develop, for research purposes, new ways of classifying mental disorders based on behavioral dimensions and neurobiological measures."[39] RDoC was introduced to address limitations of categorical DSM and ICD diagnoses. Such diagnostic categories, although reliable for diagnosing psychiatric disorders for research studies, ignore the inherent overlap among symptoms across diagnostic categories and the variability of symptom presentation within disorders. A classification system that is based on objective brain characteristics accurately measured in individual patients may address some of these concerns. As mentioned earlier, individual-specific analysis of fMRI data has shown potential in identifying biomarkers for various clinical symptoms, including both global and dimensional symptoms.[25,27] Classifying patients according to these imaging markers may lead to novel categories of disordered brain circuits that are more closely related to nervous system disorders and that better inform treatment strategies.

POTENTIAL IMPLICATIONS FOR DRUG DEVELOPMENT

In recent years, many pharmaceutical companies have allocated additional resources to nonpsychiatric drug development while reducing resources from psychiatric drug development efforts. Given the limited efficacy of current treatment with psychiatric drugs, reduction in the investment of drugs for mental disorder creates an unmet need.[40] The lack of validated biomarkers is arguably one of the largest roadblocks in psychiatric drug development. This situation might be improved by individualized psychoradiology. With the advent of individual-specific neuroimage analysis, it is now feasible to follow individual patients longitudinally to capture brain features that track symptom fluctuations over time, which may be key in revealing biologically meaningful markers for psychiatric disorders. Some recent studies have already explored individual-specific functional analysis in healthy individuals over a long period of time.[41,42] For example, Poldrack and colleagues[42] investigated the brain connectivity of a healthy individual over 532 days. They found several dynamic functional connectivity patterns over the 18-month time frame, such as the observation that dorsal attention, somatomotor, and visual networks were highly variable across scanning sessions. In psychoradiology, similar longitudinal examinations paired with individual-specific functional analysis would lay the foundation for discovering biomarkers sensitive to symptom fluctuations, which would in turn lead to accurate patient stratification and improve the efficiency of clinical trials for drug development.

FINAL REMARKS, FUTURE CONSIDERATIONS, AND SUBSEQUENT GOALS

The current state of nosologic development in psychiatry limits the ability of investigators to use psychoradiological measures to individualize patient care. Individual-specific analysis, as opposed to case-control designs and group-level analysis, can address many of the concerns with the current methods of investigation. Moreover, by using longitudinal studies and biologically homogenous patient populations, potential findings will provide higher clinical value for each patient, identify subtypes of patients for different interventions, and quantify the utility of the provided treatments, potentially expediting the process of finding novel biomarkers and therapeutic targets to advance, treatment development and clinical practice to relieve suffering of patients with highly prevalent psychiatric disorders.

DISCLOSURE

The authors have nothing to disclose.

REFERENCES

1. Huang X, Gong Q, Sweeney JA, et al. Progress in psychoradiology, the clinical application of psychiatric neuroimaging. Br J Radiol 2019;92(1101): 20181000.
2. Port JD. Diagnosis of attention deficit hyperactivity disorder by using MR imaging and radiomics: a potential tool for clinicians. Radiology 2018;287(2): 631–2.
3. Sun H, Chen Y, Huang Q, et al. Psychoradiologic utility of MR imaging for diagnosis of attention deficit hyperactivity disorder: a radiomics analysis. Radiology 2018;287(2):620–30.
4. Lui S, Deng W, Huang X, et al. Association of cerebral deficits with clinical symptoms in antipsychotic-naive first-episode schizophrenia: an optimized voxel-based morphometry and resting state functional connectivity study. Am J Psychiatry 2009;166(2):196–205.
5. Tregellas J. Connecting brain structure and function in schizophrenia. Am J Psychiatry 2009;166(2): 134–6.
6. Gong Q, Lui S, Sweeney JA. A selective review of cerebral abnormalities in patients with first-episode schizophrenia before and after treatment. Am J Psychiatry 2016;173(3):232–43.
7. Lui S, Zhou XJ, Sweeney JA, et al. Psychoradiology: the frontier of neuroimaging in psychiatry. Radiology 2016;281(2):357–72.
8. Cuthbert BN, Insel TR. Toward the future of psychiatric diagnosis: the seven pillars of RDoC. BMC Med 2013;11:126.
9. Frances A. The new crisis of confidence in psychiatric diagnosis. Ann Intern Med 2013;159(3):221–2.
10. Miller MB, Van Horn JD. Individual variability in brain activations associated with episodic retrieval: a role for large-scale databases. Int J Psychophysiol 2007; 63(2):205–13.
11. Van Horn JD, Grafton ST, Miller MB. Individual variability in brain activity: a nuisance or an opportunity? Brain Imaging Behav 2008;2(4):327–34.
12. Braga RM, Buckner RL. Parallel interdigitated distributed networks within the individual estimated by intrinsic functional connectivity. Neuron 2017; 95(2):457–71.e5.
13. Fisher AJ, Medaglia JD, Jeronimus BF. Lack of group-to-individual generalizability is a threat to human subjects research. Proc Natl Acad Sci U S A 2018;115(27):E6106–15.
14. Dubois J, Adolphs R. Building a science of individual differences from fMRI. Trends Cogn Sci 2016; 20(6):425–43.
15. Bennett CM, Miller MB. How reliable are the results from functional magnetic resonance imaging? Ann N Y Acad Sci 2010;1191:133–55.
16. Fernandez G, Specht K, Weis S, et al. Intrasubject reproducibility of presurgical language lateralization and mapping using fMRI. Neurology 2003;60(6): 969–75.
17. Harrington G, Buonocore M, Farias ST. Intrasubject reproducibility of functional MR imaging activation in language tasks. AJNR Am J Neuroradiol 2006; 27(4):938–44.
18. Elliott ML, Knodt AR, Ireland D, et al. What is the test-retest reliability of common task-fMRI measures? New empirical evidence and a meta-analysis. bioRxiv 2019;681700.
19. Wang D, Buckner RL, Fox MD, et al. Parcellating cortical functional networks in individuals. Nat Neurosci 2015;18(12):1853.
20. Finn ES, Shen X, Scheinost D, et al. Functional connectome fingerprinting: identifying individuals using patterns of brain connectivity. Nat Neurosci 2015; 18(11):1664–71.
21. Tavor I, Parker Jones O, Mars RB, et al. Task-free MRI predicts individual differences in brain activity during task performance. Science 2016;352(6282): 216–20.
22. Mueller S, Wang D, Fox MD, et al. Individual variability in functional connectivity architecture of the human brain. Neuron 2013;77(3):586–95.
23. Li M, Wang D, Ren J, et al. Performing group-level functional image analyses based on homologous functional regions mapped in individuals. PLoS Biol 2019;17(3):e2007032.
24. Kong R, Li J, Orban C, et al. Spatial topography of individual-specific cortical networks predicts human cognition, personality, and emotion. Cereb Cortex 2018;29(6):2533–51.
25. Wang D, Li M, Wang M, et al. Individual-specific functional connectivity markers track dimensional and categorical features of psychotic illness. Mol Psychiatry 2018;1.
26. Baker JT, Holmes AJ, Masters GA, et al. Disruption of cortical association networks in schizophrenia and psychotic bipolar disorder. JAMA Psychiatry 2014;71(2):109–18.
27. Brennan BP, Wang D, Li M, et al. Use of an individual-level approach to identify cortical connectivity biomarkers in obsessive-compulsive disorder. Biol Psychiatry Cogn Neurosci Neuroimaging 2019; 4(1):27–38.
28. Leucht S, Hierl S, Kissling W, et al. Putting the efficacy of psychiatric and general medicine medication into perspective: review of meta-analyses. Br J Psychiatry 2012;200(2):97–106.
29. O'Reardon JP, Solvason HB, Janicak PG, et al. Efficacy and safety of transcranial magnetic stimulation in the acute treatment of major depression: a

multisite randomized controlled trial. Biol Psychiatry 2007;62(11):1208–16.

30. Trevizol AP, Shiozawa P, Cook IA, et al. Transcranial magnetic stimulation for obsessive-compulsive disorder: an updated systematic review and meta-analysis. J ECT 2016;32(4):262–6.

31. Fregni F, Pascual-Leone A. Technology insight: noninvasive brain stimulation in neurology-perspectives on the therapeutic potential of rTMS and tDCS. Nat Clin Pract Neurol 2007;3(7):383–93.

32. Luber BM, Davis S, Bernhardt E, et al. Using neuroimaging to individualize TMS treatment for depression: toward a new paradigm for imaging-guided intervention. Neuroimage 2017;148:1–7.

33. Padberg F, George MS. Repetitive transcranial magnetic stimulation of the prefrontal cortex in depression. Exp Neurol 2009;219(1):2–13.

34. Fox MD, Liu H, Pascual-Leone A. Identification of reproducible individualized targets for treatment of depression with TMS based on intrinsic connectivity. Neuroimage 2013;66:151–60.

35. Weigand A, Horn A, Caballero R, et al. Prospective validation that subgenual connectivity predicts antidepressant efficacy of transcranial magnetic stimulation sites. Biol Psychiatry 2018;84(1):28–37.

36. Drysdale AT, Grosenick L, Downar J, et al. Resting-state connectivity biomarkers define neurophysiological subtypes of depression. Nat Med 2017; 23(1):28–38.

37. Sun H, Lui S, Yao L, et al. Two patterns of white matter abnormalities in medication-naive patients with first-episode schizophrenia revealed by diffusion tensor imaging and cluster analysis. JAMA Psychiatry 2015;72(7):678–86.

38. McTeague LM, Lang PJ. The anxiety spectrum and the reflex physiology of defense: from circumscribed fear to broad distress. Depress Anxiety 2012;29(4): 264–81.

39. Sanislow CA, Pine DS, Quinn KJ, et al. Developing constructs for psychopathology research: research domain criteria. J Abnorm Psychol 2010;119(4): 631–9.

40. Insel T, Voon V, Nye J, et al. Innovative solutions to novel drug development in mental health. Neurosci Biobehav Rev 2013;37(10):2438–44.

41. Laumann TO, Gordon EM, Adeyemo B, et al. Functional system and areal organization of a highly sampled individual human brain. Neuron 2015; 87(3):657–70.

42. Poldrack RA, Laumann TO, Koyejo O, et al. Long-term neural and physiological phenotyping of a single human. Nat Commun 2015;6:8885.

Psychoradiological Biomarkers for Psychopharmaceutical Effects

Anouk Schrantee, PhD[a], Henricus Gerardus Ruhé, MD, PhD[b,c],
Liesbeth Reneman, MD, PhD[a,*]

KEYWORDS

- Psychoradiology • Predictive imaging biomarkers • Treatment response • Antidepressants
- Stimulants

KEY POINTS

- The literature on psychoradiological imaging biomarkers that target treatment response is in general highly heterogeneous, with underpowered studies and a large amount of variation in techniques and analysis approaches.
- The most replicated finding at present is the relation of antidepressant treatment response to hippocampal (subfield) size.
- Rigorous validation and replication studies are needed, with emphasis on multimodal and noninvasive imaging biomarkers, obtained in large-scale consortia.

INTRODUCTION

Despite advances in pharmacology, not all psychiatric patients respond favorably to drugs. Currently, psychiatric medication is prescribed based on a "trial-and-error" method. This means patients have to deal with nonresponse, side effects, and adverse events. For example, for major depression, only approximately 30% to 50% of patients will have full remission of symptoms after first-line treatment, with cumulative remission rates of approximately 67% after 4 trials of different antidepressants. In some instances, the evidence for pharmacologic treatment is also lacking (eg, applied in a specific disease or age range). However, progress in the understanding of disease mechanism and drug action is opening up opportunities to match therapies to patient populations and thus pave the way toward personalized medicine. The concept of personalized medicine, also called precision medicine, that is, prevention and treatment strategies that take individual variability into account, is not new: blood typing, for instance, has been used to guide blood transfusions for more than a century. This personalized approach heavily relies on biomarkers that take into account an individual's genes, environment, and lifestyle. An algorithm weighing all these factors then provides the physician with data regarding the best medical intervention for a specific patient. Recent developments of large-scale biological databases, characterization of patients (using proteomics, metabolomics, genomics, and radiomics) and computational tools for analyzing large datasets have dramatically improved the possibility of applying this concept.

Disclosure Statement: The authors have nothing to disclose.
[a] Department of Radiology and Nuclear Medicine, Amsterdam UMC, Academic Medical Center, Meibergdreef 9, Amsterdam 1105AZ, the Netherlands; [b] Department of Psychiatry, Radboud University Medical Centre, Reinier Postlaan 4, 6525 GC, Nijmegen, the Netherlands; [c] Donders Institute for Brain, Cognition and Behavior, Radboud University, Montessorilaan 3, 6525 HR, Nijmegen, the Netherlands
* Corresponding author.
E-mail address: L.Reneman@amsterdamumc.nl

Neuroimag Clin N Am 30 (2020) 53–63
https://doi.org/10.1016/j.nic.2019.09.006
1052-5149/20/© 2019 The Authors. Published by Elsevier Inc.

For example, personalized medicine is already revolutionizing cancer treatment, in which treatments are tailored to a tumor's genomic profile.

The application of personalized medicine to psychiatry, however, is more challenging. Yet psychiatric disorders are responsible for immense personal, social, and financial burden. Indeed, the lifetime prevalence of various psychiatric disorders among the population is approximately 30% to 40%. In contrast to cancer, there is no biological or histological test for definitive psychiatric diagnoses, because of the inaccessibility of the human brain. The diagnosis is based on a combination of symptoms alone, by standard nosology, as reflected in diagnostic manuals, such as the *Diagnostic and Statistical Manual of Mental Disorders* (DSM) or the *International Classification of Diseases*. The emerging field of psychoradiology, pioneered by Gong and colleagues,[1–3] could provide biomarkers based on objective tests in support of the diagnostic classifications, as in other parts of medicine. Because of its noninvasive nature, it has great potential to revolutionize clinical psychiatry. In particular, this is plausible based on the hypothesis for psychoradiology by Gong and colleagues,[1] who proposed a "brain structure-function-behavioral conjunction" theory in which brain structural alteration leads to clinical syndrome, likely due to the conjunction impact of the impaired functional connectivity.[3–5] Progress in related work has benefitted from methodological advances for detecting the psychopathologies at individual patient level,[6,7] as Dr Hesheng Liu and his colleagues from Harvard Medical School suggest in Hesheng Liu and colleagues' article "Individual-Specific Analysis for Psychoradiology," in this issue.

Diagnostic and Predictive Biomarkers

As outlined by the Health Research Directorate of the EU, a biomarker is a biological characteristic, which can be molecular, anatomical, physiological, or biochemical in nature. These characteristics can be measured and evaluated objectively. Biomarkers are either diagnostic markers that index biological characteristics associated with health or disease, or predictive, reflecting a process associated with therapeutic response. Psychoradiology could satisfy these goals, because it can provide several molecular, anatomical, physiological, and biochemical characteristics of the living human brain. For instance, PET, single-photon emission computed tomography (SPECT) and the more recently developed technique pharmacologic MR imaging (phMR imaging) are used for molecular imaging of the brain. Anatomical

characteristics can be obtained using detailed structural imaging, physiological characteristics using functional MR imaging (fMR imaging) and perfusion imaging (eg, arterial spin labeling [ASL]), and biochemical characteristics using MR spectroscopy (MRS). These psychoradiological characteristics might be part of a panel of tests that also include, for example, genetic, peripheral blood-based, or cognitive tests.

Here, we focus on predictive psychoradiological biomarkers for pharmacotherapy as one subset of potential biomarkers in psychiatry. The main challenges of predictive psychoradiological biomarkers for psychiatric disorders are discussed and current advances outlined. The article concludes with some future directions for the translation of psychoradiological characteristics into clinically useful biomarkers.

CHALLENGES OF PSYCHORADIOLOGICAL BIOMARKERS FOR PSYCHIATRIC DISORDERS

In the field of psychiatric research, most studies use case-control designs in an attempt to uncover *diagnostic* biomarkers. However, to develop *predictive* biomarkers, studies using stratified sampling of patients are needed. In fact, Abi-Dargham and Horga[8] argue that the lack of personalized treatment in psychiatry is due to several challenges associated with discovering imaging biomarkers for psychiatric disorders, as opposed to, for example, cancer biomarkers. The first main challenge is the lack of a "gold standard" or definitive biological or histologic tests for psychiatric diagnoses. This complicates the validation of the biomarker, which requires correlative analysis of the psychoradiological characteristics against the definitive outcome. Currently, longitudinal follow-up is frequently needed to establish a final diagnosis. However, diagnostic information obtained from longitudinal follow-up is complex because it can be confounded by epiphenomenal consequences of the illness or its treatment. This precludes a direct association between the psychoradiological biomarker and brain-based phenotypes.

The second main challenge is that the pathologic features of psychiatric disease may be subtle and surface in only specific situations or under a certain cognitive load. Indeed, psychiatric disorders have been shown to be polygenic; usually the penetrance of a single gene variant is low, because the pathologic feature of that variant will only show as an added effect to the overall phenotype. Symptoms that we associate with psychiatric disorders may emerge only if the amount of (pathologic) gene variants exceeds a certain threshold and/or these variants interact with negative environmental factors. The value of psychiatric biomarkers might therefore be dependent on studying these disorders (or individuals) under specific circumstances or conditions. To this end, challenge-paradigms have been used, and are now regarded an essential tool for the development of biomarkers. The paradigms could, for example, be task-based or pharmacologic assessments that challenge the systems or network affected in the disorder.

Some other challenges include that for PET/SPECT not all neurotransmitter systems can be currently imaged and that the development of novel tracers takes time. Furthermore, the neuroimaging field rewards novelty over replication, which explains the paucity of replicated findings, despite being essential for validation of a biomarker. Finally, a practical challenge in the development of psychoradiological biomarkers is the costs of the scans: in the United States, MR imaging scans cost approximately $600 per hour in academic centers and up to $1000 per hour for commercial centers, and PET scans range from $3000 to $5000 per scan.

CURRENT POTENTIAL PREDICTIVE PSYCHORADIOLOGICAL BIOMARKERS FOR PSYCHOPHARMACEUTICAL EFFECTS

Notwithstanding these challenges, some potential psychoradiological biomarkers have already been identified. In this article, we summarize studies aiming to establish markers of disease progression, or response to interventions (ie, predictive biomarkers). We do so for 3 prevalent psychiatric diseases and the most prescribed psychotropic medications in adults and children/adolescents, namely antidepressants for major depressive disorder (MDD), anxiolytics for anxiety disorders (ADs) and stimulants for attention-deficit/hyperactivity disorder (ADHD).[9,10] This overview is restricted to studies addressing pharmacologic treatment only. Furthermore, studies using predictive neurophysiological biomarkers (eg, electroencephalogram) are beyond the scope of this review.

Major Depressive Disorder

Major depression is the most prevalent psychiatric disorder in adults and children in the Western world, resulting in a heavy global disease burden. First-line, evidence-based treatments for adults and children and adolescents with MDD include structured psychotherapies (eg, cognitive behavioral therapy and interpersonal psychotherapy) and antidepressant medications. Selective serotonin reuptake inhibitors (SSRIs) are most commonly prescribed, of which only fluoxetine is registered for treatment of depression and AD in children (aged 8 years and older). However, approximately 30% to 40% of patients fail to respond, and this rate is even higher in children. Because treatment efficacy only can be reliably assessed after 6 to 12 weeks of treatment, continuation of an ineffective treatment to establish treatment response'nonresponse prolongs patient suffering related to depressive symptoms and reinforces the general perception of patients that there is nothing they can do to overcome the depressive disorder (ie, facilitating demotivation).

Using structural MR imaging, a meta-analysis showed that a smaller right hippocampal volume was a significant predictor of poorer treatment response in MDD.[11] Although subsequent studies suggest that lower total hippocampal volume was largely explained by brain atrophy,[12] larger tail and subiculum volumes have been shown to be predictive of symptom reduction.[12,13] It is worth noting that longer illness duration also has been associated with smaller hippocampal volumes,[14] but this appeared to be independent of the positive relation between larger tail volumes and remission.[12] This is in line with a large body of research implicating volumetric changes to the hippocampus in the etiology of MDD.

A meta-analysis of 20 functional PET with fludeoxyglucose ([18F]FDG-PET) and MR imaging studies found that higher pretreatment activity in the anterior cingulate cortex is predictive of a higher likelihood of improvement,[15] whereas higher pretreatment activation in the insula and striatum is associated with higher likelihood of a poorer clinical response. However, this meta-analysis also pointed out the substantial heterogeneity between studies, in terms of design, patient groups, and tasks used to elicit functional activation. A recent systematic review on functional connectivity studies addressing network dynamics in response to antidepressants reported that treatment response is consistently associated with increased connectivity between frontal and limbic brain regions (possibly resulting in greater inhibitory control over neural circuits that process emotions).[16] However, the most recent study found the reverse; that is, negative functional connectivity with the subcallosal cingulate cortex was associated with remission to medication, whereas positive functional connectivity scores were associated with treatment failure.[17] Interestingly, the remission and treatment failure to cognitive behavioral therapy (CBT) was predicted by exactly opposite functional connectivity scores.

Molecular imaging studies furthermore found that higher pretreatment availability and greater occupancy of serotonin transporter (SERT) correlated with improved treatment response in the short term, using both SPECT and PET.[18,19] However, 3 studies did not find such a relation,[20–22] and another study only demonstrated this relation in a specific genotype.[23] A review focusing on MRS concluded that there is strong evidence that changes in glutamate, N-acetylaspartate, and choline demonstrate a good correlation with treatment response to pharmacotherapy.[24] However, later studies reported conflicting results. For example, greater increases in gamma-aminobutyric acid (GABA) levels were found to be significantly associated with clinical response after a week of citalopram treatment, whereas no association with glutamate was found.[25] In contrast, another study found no predictive properties of GABA but did report that decreased occipital glutamate may be a biomarker of antidepressant response.[26] Furthermore, a study at 7T investigating treatment response to the novel antidepressant ketamine found no association with pretreatment glutamate levels.[27] The investigators report that the effects of the medication were smaller than the measurement sensitivity ($\sim$8%), which might explain the variable results found at 3T, which has even lower sensitivity.

Whereas research on predictive biomarkers for adults is starting to emerge, this is limited evidence for children and adolescents. Moreover, clinical indications suggest that SSRI exposure during adolescence may lead to negative outcomes that are not seen in adult patients. For instance, the most serious side effect associated with SSRIs prescribed to children is increased suicide risk,[28] which led to a black box warning from the Food and Drug Administration (FDA) and European Medicines Agency (EMA) in 2004. A small study in 13 adolescents with MDD found that the greater reduction of anxiety (but not depression) symptoms was associated with higher pretreatment fMR imaging striatal activity and lower medial prefrontal cortex (PFC) activity, in both CBT and CBT + SSRI-treated individuals.[29] In 19 medication-naïve depressed adolescents, fluoxetine-induced decreases in both limbic and frontal activation did not correspond with clinical treatment response.[30] Cullen and colleagues[31] found that treatment response to SSRIs was associated with increased amygdala functional connectivity with right frontal cortex, and decreased amygdala connectivity with right precuneus and right posterior cingulate cortex in 13 medication-naïve adolescents with MDD/AD.

In summary, the current literature on psychoradiological imaging predictors that target treatment response and remission in MDD is highly heterogeneous, with generally underpowered studies and a large amount of variation in techniques and analysis approaches. At present, the most replicated finding is the relation of treatment response to hippocampal (subfield) size. In adolescents, most fMR imaging studies focused on aberrant amygdala activity, but found conflicting results, as in adult studies, possibly reflecting medication status, comorbid disorders, but also possibly reflecting technical difficulties acquiring fMR imaging signal in this area.[32] Other frontolimbic regions, including the prefrontal cortex, anterior cingulate cortex, and insula are other regions of interest in the discovery of additional predictive psychoradiological biomarkers for MDD,[33] as well as the intrinsic functional brain connectivity including greater within-network (default mode network) and between-network (default mode network and executive control network) connectivity, higher connectivity of the hippocampus with the limbic network and somatomotor network, and lower connectivity of the thalamus with the limbic network.[34]

Anxiety

ADs, including generalized anxiety disorder (GAD), panic disorder (PAD), social anxiety disorder (SAD), and simple phobias are (together with MDD) the most common psychiatric illnesses experienced, affecting an estimated 18% of people in the United States. Although both obsessive compulsive disorder and posttraumatic stress disorder have been classified as ADs in the past, they have been removed from the category in the DSM-5. The most prescribed pharmacologic treatment consists of SSRIs and serotonin and norepinephrine reuptake inhibitors, but for example, only 12% of patients with PD were in full remission after 5 years.[35] Moreover, 40% to 45% of youth with AD do not achieve remission (or a substantial reduction in symptoms) following treatment. Although most of the neuroimaging biomarker research in AD has applied psychotherapy (as this is the first-line treatment) rather than pharmacologic interventions, a few psychoradiological studies have been designed to explore brain markers of pharmacologic response in AD, as reviewed by Maron and Nutt.[36]

Predictive effects of structural measures on treatment response in AD have not been systematically evaluated as in MDD. However, small studies in patients with PD demonstrated that changes in total gray matter volume after remission were correlated with changes in clinical scores,[37] and that white matter micro-structural integrity increased in the right uncinate fasciculus and left fronto-occipital fasciculus after remission in patients with PD on escitalopram treatment.[38]

The most recent systematic review in AD[39] indicated increased reactivity in neural networks subserving threat processing (eg, amygdala, insula (dorsal) anterior cingulate cortex (ACC) and PFC/orbitofrontal cortex) as a potential biomarker with predictive value for treatment response. For instance, in patients with GAD, higher pretreatment fMR imaging ACC and amygdala activity is associated with stronger reductions in anxiety and worry symptoms after 8 weeks of treatment with venlafaxine.[40,41] In contrast, a small sample of patients with SAD who did not respond to SSRIs demonstrated higher regional cerebral blood flow (CBF) ([^{99m}Tc]HMPAO SPECT) in the left temporal cortex and the left midfrontal regions at baseline as compared with responders.[42] In another study, amygdala-frontal CBF ([^{15}O]H$_2$O PET) response to a public-speaking task differed between responders and nonresponders to SSRIs and placebo in a large randomized clinical trial of patients with SAD.[43] Finally, treatment response to tiagabine, an anticonvulsant drug prescribed off-label for AD, was inversely correlated with pretreatment cerebral metabolic rate of glucose uptake ([^{18}F]FDG-PET) within the ventromedial PFC in 12 patients with generalized SAD.[44]

Although the literature in AD predominantly focused on adults, an fMR imaging study in pediatric AD found that less recruitment of the dorsal ACC and dorsomedial PFC during emotional processing predicted a greater reduction in anxiety symptoms following SSRI treatment (as well as CBT),[45] similar to a prior study that found that greater activation in prefrontal regions (involved in social signals of threat) predicted better response to sertraline in anxious youth.[46]

In sum, the current literature on psychoradiological imaging predictors that target treatment response and remission in AD is limited, possibly because psychotherapy is often the first-line treatment of choice rather than pharmacologic interventions (Table 1).

Attention-Deficit/Hyperactivity Disorder

Psychostimulants, including methylphenidate (MPH) and dexamphetamine, are generally considered first-line management for the core symptoms of ADHD. Although stimulants are successful in reducing ADHD symptoms, it has been estimated that 10% to 30% of patients with ADHD do not respond adequately to MPH.[47] In contrast to MDD and AD, substantially more imaging research has been performed in children with

Table 1 Predictive biomarkers of nonresponse in MDD and AD (as indicated by level I evidence [systematic reviews and meta-analysis])	
Structural imaging	↓ Volume of hippocampus (MDD adults)
CBF	↓ Baseline CBF in ACC (MDD adults)
task-fMR imaging	↓ Reactivity in amygdala, insula, (dorsal) ACC and PFC/OFC (MDD and AD children and adults)
rs-fMR imaging	↓ Functional connectivity between frontal and limbic brain regions (MDD adults)

Abbreviations: ↓, indicates a reduction; ACC, anterior cingulate cortex; AD, anxiety disorder; CBF, cerebral blood flow; fMR imaging; functional magnetic resonance imaging; MDD, major depressive disorder; PFC/OFC, prefrontal cortex/orbitofrontal cortex; rs-fMRI, restingstate-fMRI.

ADHD compared with adults. Therefore, studies in this section are grouped only by neuroimaging measure used and not by age.

Structural MR imaging findings in children with ADHD include a thinner pretreatment left medial PFC[48] and smaller corpus callosum,[49] reversed caudate asymmetry and smaller retro-callosal parietal-occipital white matter volumes,[50] as well as smaller posterior cerebellar lobes[51] in nonresponders. Moreno and colleagues[52] found a correlation between caudate nucleus and nucleus accumbens volumes and clinical and neuropsychological improvement after MPH treatment in 27 medication-naïve children with ADHD. This is in line with a meta-analysis reporting that reduced basal ganglia volume is the most prominent and replicable structural abnormality in ADHD.[53]

Most studies, however, have used invasive imaging with PET and SPECT, assessing dopamine (DA) transporter and D$_1$ and D$_2$ receptor availability, along with brain perfusion studies. Pediatric nonresponders to MPH seem to have different patterns of CBF ([^{99m}Tc]HMPAO SPECT) in the frontal-striatal circuitry and the posterior attentional system.[54] In addition, children with ADHD who displayed higher off-medication CBF ([^{15}O] H$_2$O PET) in the midbrain, posterior cerebellum, and middle frontal gyrus were less likely to respond to MPH on current ADHD rating scales.[55] Similarly in adults, a large retrospective study in 157 patients demonstrated that prefrontal CBF change to a sustained attention task was a highly sensitive and specific predictor of response to stimulants, with prefrontal pole activation predicting adverse responses and deactivation predicting good responses.[56] As for the dopamine system, high DAT binding was associated with poor response to stimulant treatment (and presence of homozygosity of the 10-repeat allele on the DAT-1 gene) in a small sample of children.[57] It was further observed in children that the lower the baseline striatal D_2 levels ([^{123}I]IBZM SPECT), the lower the response rate.[58] In adults, 2 studies found, contrary to results in children, that medication-naïve patients with high striatal DAT availability ([^{99}mTc]TRODAT SPECT) responded better to therapy with MPH than those with low DAT availability.[59,60]

A surprisingly small number of studies have investigated the relation between brain function and treatment response, despite the wealth of fMR imaging studies on the effect of stimulants on, for example, inhibition tasks. However, one study focusing on functional connectivity in children found that a good response to MPH is associated with reduced ventral striatal connectivity with the inferior frontal cortices when compared with poor responders.[61]

In sum, very few studies using nonionizing techniques have investigated treatment response in ADHD, and all have been in children. This might be due to the generally high treatment response of approximately 70%. However, this does not mean that we cannot improve treatment outcomes using personalized medicine, because many patients experience side effects, and therefore adherence can be low, especially in adults (Table 2). ADHD patients can be divided into several subgroups based on the different manifestations of EEG, which could predict their different treatment outcomes.[62] For the biomarker of brain volume detected by MRI, the degree of

hippocampal subfields volume reduction in schizophrenia was associated with the dosage of antipsychotics.[63] The possible use of biomarkers for dose optimization would be beneficial in clinical practice.

FUTURE DIRECTIONS FOR PREDICTIVE PSYCHORADIOLOGICAL BIOMARKERS FOR PHARMACEUTICAL TREATMENT EFFECTS

None of the potential psychoradiological biomarkers reviewed are yet of sufficiently established clinical utility to inform the selection of a specific pharmacologic compound for an individual patient. Most studies described have been conducted in small samples or had clear shortcomings in their clinical design and treatment outcome assessment (which is beyond the scope of this article to review). Nevertheless, there is strong consensus that advanced multimodal approaches, combining neuroimaging, genetic, and proteomic techniques, should contribute to discovery of novel treatment predictors in psychiatric disorders. Progress so far has been sufficient to warrant enthusiasm, in which application of neuroimaging-based biomarkers would represent a paradigm shift and modernization of psychiatric practice. Therefore, the development of clinically useful biomarkers should be a top priority of mental health research, as recognized by the National Institute of Mental Health (NIMH), FDA, and EMA. The recently developed NIMH Research Domain Criteria (RDoC) Framework may aid in development of psychoradiological biomarkers by classifying mental disorders based on dimensions of observable behavior and neurobiological mechanisms, rather than symptoms alone. Furthermore, RDoC also suggests that several circuit-based behavioral dimensions may be shared across psychiatric disorders. However, it is important to note that the transition to RDoC will take time, and the question arises if and when treatment planning should be adjusted to this new framework. Moreover, it remains to be established whether RDoC parameters will be the ideal way forward to categorize or even dimensionally evaluate psychiatric patients.

Validation and Replication

Because the ultimate goal of psychoradiological biomarkers is to aid clinical practice and thus provide useful information over and above symptomatic and sociodemographic data, the next step is to validate potential biomarkers rigorously. Validation would entail demonstration that a biomarker can perform effectively and reproducibly and can facilitate improvement of treatment outcome or

Table 2 Predictive biomarkers of nonresponse to MPH in ADHD	
Structural imaging	↓ Volume of caudate, cerebellum, corpus callosum, prefrontal cortex (children)
CBF	↑ CBF in midbrain, posterior cerebellum, and middle frontal gyrus, ACC, the left claustrum, and the right (children and adults)
DAT	↓ Striatal DAT in adults, ↑ DAT in children

Abbreviations: ↓, indicates a reduction; ↑, indicates a increase; ACC, anterior cingulate cortex; ADHD, attention-deficit/hyperactivity disorder; CBF, cerebral blood flow; DAT, dopamine transporter; MPH, methylphenidate.

prediction of prognosis in individual patients. Especially the latter is difficult. What is needed now is external validation of potential psychoradiological biomarkers in independent clinical samples of sufficient size and description in terms of their predictive value, sensitivity and specificity for a desired outcome. Although a biomarker would typically have sensitivity and specificity values higher than 90%, a modest predictive value might be clinically impactful, if the standard care is based on an arbitrary decision between 2 comparable alternatives. Then, longitudinal randomized designs are needed to quantify the clinical utility of the biomarkers, by demonstrating that in a biomarker-guided treatment arm versus a nonguided arm, their use is associated with a reduction in morbidity and improvement in quality of life. An example of a study evaluating the use of changes in face recognition in the first 2 weeks of antidepressant use in MDD as a predictive biomarker is the PReDiCT-trial, in which a validated algorithm is currently being tested in a pan-European multicenter randomized controlled trial.[64]

To generate a larger pool of potential biomarkers, it is essential that obligatory replication using identical paradigms in well-powered studies needs to be accepted as the norm. For instance, whereas amygdala activity in response to emotional stimuli was reported as a potential fMR imaging biomarker predicting symptom reduction in MDD and AD, it was found to have low within-subject reproducibility.[65] In addition, it is necessary to familiarize ourselves with the limits of our imaging techniques. As mentioned previously,[27] the expected change in the physiologic parameter of interest should be large enough as to overcome the intrinsic variability of our measurement. Biomarker development requires a priori designed, large-scale multisite treatment efficacy, notably randomized controlled trials with coordinated, pre-planned analysis plans that include independent validation, rather than post hoc sharing of data sets acquired from multiple studies with differing goals. To this purpose, reproducibility across sites should be tested using quality assurance tests on scanners as well as specific (automated) analysis software for data processing.

Multimodality

Given the multimodal nature of findings, it appears most promising to increase single-subject prediction accuracies by integrating biomarkers from neuroimaging data, genetic, and clinical information. Combining these modalities does not only hold the promise of more accurate predictions, but also enables the identification of the most efficient, nonredundant set of predictors. There is a definite lack of studies integrating clinical, genetic, and imaging information using machine learning approaches.[66] For instance, Whitfield-Gabrieli and colleagues[67] integrated clinical parameters and neuroimaging markers in patients with SAD (rs-fMR imaging and DTI), and predicted response to CBT substantially better than a current clinician-administrated measure of disease severity. Support vector machine classification was 84.6% accurate for predicting MPH response in ADHD using pretreatment demographic, clinical questionnaire, environmental, neuropsychological, neuroimaging, and genetic data,[68] although the neuroimaging measures were not the most differentiating subset of features. Another approach with potential would be normative modeling; an approach, which unlike machine learning approaches that use clustering to categorize cohorts, aims to map variation within the sample. In that way, it allows for parsing heterogeneity, while still allowing predictions at a patient-specific level.[69]

Noninvasive Biomarkers

Predictive biomarkers should not only be reliable and reproducible, but they should ideally also be as noninvasive as possible. Therefore, psychoradiological biomarkers ideally also should not make use of radiation or external contrast agents. For example, well-validated task-fMR imaging paradigms could be used to target specific cognitive functions or behavioral patterns that are aberrant in specific disorders or across RDoCs to discover biomarkers.[70] A more recent noninvasive technique is phMR imaging, which is based on the principle that neurotransmitter-specific drug challenges evoke regional changes in neurovascular coupling and resultant changes in brain hemodynamics. We have shown that phMR imaging may be a suitable alternative to assess the 5-HT and DA system,[71–73] although the field still has to establish itself in terms of sensitivity and specificity compared with conventional methods, such as PET and SPECT.[74] Nevertheless, by using phMR imaging in clinical trials, we were able to demonstrate important age-dependent changes induced by the SSRI fluoxetine and MPH on the developing brain.[75,76] Thus, in the near future phMR imaging could become the technique of choice to investigate differences in predictive biomarkers regarding treatment outcome across the life span, as there are notable differences in the neurobiological correlates of patients in different age cohorts (despite similarities in the clinical picture and longitudinal course of psychiatric disorders in children and adults). In addition to phMR imaging, MRS could also be an interesting noninvasive imaging modality to aid in psychiatric biomarker research. Application of MRS at high field strengths and advances in acquisition protocols have improved MRS data significantly over the past decade.[77] Furthermore, MRS can directly measure concentrations of 2 of the most important neurotransmitters in the brain, that is, glutamate and GABA. These measurements are not based on hemodynamic measurements and are therefore less influenced by cardiovascular changes that can be induced by comorbid illness, medication, or age. In sum, the literature on psychoradiological imaging biomarkers that target treatment response is in general highly heterogeneous, with underpowered studies and a large amount of variation in techniques and analysis approaches. The most replicated finding at present is the relation of antidepressant treatment response to hippocampal (subfield) size. But with rigorous validation and replication studies, with emphasis on multimodal and noninvasive imaging biomarkers, obtained in large-scale consortia, psychoradiological biomarkers for psychopharmaceutical effects have the potential to revolutionize clinical psychiatry.

ACKNOWLEDGMENTS

This work was sponsored by grant #ESTAR19210 from Eurostars and by grant #11.32050.26 from the European Research Area Network Priority Medicines for Children (Sixth Framework Programme). Dr Schrantee was supported by a Veni grant Veni (Netherlands Organisation for Scientific Research). Dr Ruhe was supported by ZonMW/NWO VENI-grant #016.126.059, the Hersenstichting Grant #2009(2)-72 and participated in an EU Horizon 2020 (SME Instrument project) grant #696802.

REFERENCES

1. Gong Q, Lui S, Sweeney JA. A selective review of cerebral abnormalities in patients with first-episode schizophrenia before and after treatment. Am J Psychiatry 2016;173:232–43.
2. Huang X, Gong Q, Sweeney JA, et al. Progress in psychoradiology, the clinical application of psychiatric neuroimaging. Br J Radiol 2019;92:20181000.
3. Lui S, Zhou XJ, Sweeney JA, et al. Psychoradiology: the frontier of neuroimaging in psychiatry. Radiology 2016;281:357–72.
4. Lui S, Deng W, Huang X, et al. Association of cerebral deficits with clinical symptoms in antipsychotic-naive first-episode schizophrenia: an optimized voxel-based morphometry and resting state functional connectivity study. Am J Psychiatry 2009;166:196–205.
5. Tregellas J. Connecting brain structure and function in schizophrenia. Am J Psychiatry 2009;166:134–6.
6. Wang D, Li M, Wang M, et al. Individual-specific functional connectivity markers track dimensional and categorical features of psychotic illness. Mol Psychiatry 2018. [Epub ahead of print].
7. Lei D, Pinaya WHL, van Amelsvoort T, et al. Detecting schizophrenia at the level of the individual: relative diagnostic value of whole-brain images, connectome-wide functional connectivity and graph-based metrics. Psychol Med 2019;1–10. [Epub ahead of print].
8. Abi-Dargham A, Horga G. The search for imaging biomarkers in psychiatric disorders. Nat Med 2016; 22:1248–55.
9. Sultan RS, Correll CU, Schoenbaum M, et al. National patterns of commonly prescribed psychotropic medications to young people. J Child Adolesc Psychopharmacol 2018;28:158–65.
10. Wittchen HU, Jacobi F, Rehm J, et al. The size and burden of mental disorders and other disorders of the brain in Europe 2010. Eur Neuropsychopharmacol 2011;21:655–79.
11. Colle R, Dupong I, Colliot O, et al. Smaller hippocampal volumes predict lower antidepressant response/remission rates in depressed patients: a meta-analysis. World J Biol Psychiatry 2018;19: 360–7.
12. Maller JJ, Broadhouse K, Rush AJ, et al. Increased hippocampal tail volume predicts depression status and remission to anti-depressant medications in major depression. Mol Psychiatry 2018;23:1737–44.
13. Hu X, Zhang L, Hu X, et al. Abnormal hippocampal subfields may be potential predictors of worse early response to antidepressant treatment in drug-naive patients with major depressive disorder. J Magn Reson Imaging 2019;49:1760–8.
14. Stratmann M, Konrad C, Kugel H, et al. Insular and hippocampal gray matter volume reductions in patients with major depressive disorder. PLoS One 2014;9:e102692.
15. Fu CH, Steiner H, Costafreda SG. Predictive neural biomarkers of clinical response in depression: a meta-analysis of functional and structural neuroimaging studies of pharmacological and psychological therapies. Neurobiol Dis 2013;52:75–83.
16. Dichter GS, Gibbs D, Smoski MJ. A systematic review of relations between resting-state functional-MRI and treatment response in major depressive disorder. J Affect Disord 2015;172:8–17.
17. Dunlop BW, Rajendra JK, Craighead WE, et al. Functional connectivity of the subcallosal cingulate cortex and differential outcomes to treatment with

cognitive-behavioral therapy or antidepressant medication for major depressive disorder. Am J Psychiatry 2017;174:533–45.

18. Kugaya A, Sanacora G, Staley JK, et al. Brain serotonin transporter availability predicts treatment response to selective serotonin reuptake inhibitors. Biol Psychiatry 2004;56:497–502.

19. Lanzenberger R, Kranz GS, Haeusler D, et al. Prediction of SSRI treatment response in major depression based on serotonin transporter interplay between median raphe nucleus and projection areas. Neuroimage 2012;63:874–81.

20. Ananth MR, DeLorenzo C, Yang J, et al. Decreased pretreatment amygdalae serotonin transporter binding in unipolar depression remitters: a prospective PET study. J Nucl Med 2018;59:665–70.

21. Meyer JH, Wilson AA, Sagrati S, et al. Serotonin transporter occupancy of five selective serotonin reuptake inhibitors at different doses: an [11C]DASB positron emission tomography study. Am J Psychiatry 2004;161:826–35.

22. Miller JM, Oquendo MA, Ogden RT, et al. Serotonin transporter binding as a possible predictor of one-year remission in major depressive disorder. J Psychiatr Res 2008;42:1137–44.

23. Ruhe HG, Ooteman W, Booij J, et al. Serotonin transporter gene promoter polymorphisms modify the association between paroxetine serotonin transporter occupancy and clinical response in major depressive disorder. Pharmacogenet Genomics 2009;19:67–76.

24. Caverzasi E, Pichiecchio A, Poloni GU, et al. Magnetic resonance spectroscopy in the evaluation of treatment efficacy in unipolar major depressive disorder: a review of the literature. Funct Neurol 2012;27:13–22.

25. Brennan BP, Admon R, Perriello C, et al. Acute change in anterior cingulate cortex GABA, but not glutamine/glutamate, mediates antidepressant response to citalopram. Psychiatry Res Neuroimaging 2017;269:9–16.

26. Abdallah CG, Niciu MJ, Fenton LR, et al. Decreased occipital cortical glutamate levels in response to successful cognitive-behavioral therapy and pharmacotherapy for major depressive disorder. Psychother Psychosom 2014;83:298–307.

27. Evans JW, Lally N, An L, et al. 7T (1)H-MRS in major depressive disorder: a Ketamine Treatment Study. Neuropsychopharmacology 2018;43:1908–14.

28. Bridge JA, Iyengar S, Salary CB, et al. Clinical response and risk for reported suicidal ideation and suicide attempts in pediatric antidepressant treatment: a meta-analysis of randomized controlled trials. JAMA 2007;297:1683–96.

29. Forbes EE, Olino TM, Ryan ND, et al. Reward-related brain function as a predictor of treatment response in adolescents with major depressive disorder. Cogn Affect Behav Neurosci 2010;10:107–18.

30. Tao R, Calley CS, Hart J, et al. Brain activity in adolescent major depressive disorder before and after fluoxetine treatment. Am J Psychiatry 2012;169:381–8.

31. Cullen KR, Klimes-Dougan B, Vu DP, et al. Neural correlates of antidepressant treatment response in adolescents with major depressive disorder. J Child Adolesc Psychopharmacol 2016;26:705–12.

32. Boubela RN, Kalcher K, Huf W, et al. fMRI measurements of amygdala activation are confounded by stimulus correlated signal fluctuation in nearby veins draining distant brain regions. Sci Rep 2015;5:10499.

33. Fonseka TM, MacQueen GM, Kennedy SH. Neuroimaging biomarkers as predictors of treatment outcome in Major Depressive Disorder. J Affect Disord 2018;233:21–35.

34. Chin Fatt CR, Jha MK, Cooper CM, et al. Effect of intrinsic patterns of functional brain connectivity in moderating antidepressant treatment response in major depression. Am J Psychiatry 2019. [Epub ahead of print].

35. Faravelli C, Paterniti S, Scarpato A. 5-year prospective, naturalistic follow-up study of panic disorder. Compr Psychiatry 1995;36:271–7.

36. Maron E, Nutt D. Biological predictors of pharmacological therapy in anxiety disorders. Dialogues Clin Neurosci 2015;17:305–17.

37. Lai CH, Wu YT. Changes in regional homogeneity of parieto-temporal regions in panic disorder patients who achieved remission with antidepressant treatment. J Affect Disord 2013;151:709–14.

38. Lai CH, Wu YT, Yu PL, et al. Improvements in white matter micro-structural integrity of right uncinate fasciculus and left fronto-occipital fasciculus of remitted first-episode medication-naive panic disorder patients. J Affect Disord 2013;150:330–6.

39. Lueken U, Zierhut KC, Hahn T, et al. Neurobiological markers predicting treatment response in anxiety disorders: a systematic review and implications for clinical application. Neurosci Biobehav Rev 2016;66:143–62.

40. Nitschke JB, Sarinopoulos I, Oathes DJ, et al. Anticipatory activation in the amygdala and anterior cingulate in generalized anxiety disorder and prediction of treatment response. Am J Psychiatry 2009;166:302–10.

41. Whalen PJ, Johnstone T, Somerville LH, et al. A functional magnetic resonance imaging predictor of treatment response to venlafaxine in generalized anxiety disorder. Biol Psychiatry 2008;63:858–63.

42. Van der Linden G, van Heerden B, Warwick J, et al. Functional brain imaging and pharmacotherapy in social phobia: single photon emission computed tomography before and after treatment with the

selective serotonin reuptake inhibitor citalopram. Prog Neuropsychopharmacol Biol Psychiatry 2000; 24:419–38.

43. Faria V, Ahs F, Appel L, et al. Amygdala-frontal couplings characterizing SSRI and placebo response in social anxiety disorder. Int J Neuropsychopharmacol 2014;17:1149–57.

44. Evans KC, Simon NM, Dougherty DD, et al. A PET study of tiagabine treatment implicates ventral medial prefrontal cortex in generalized social anxiety disorder. Neuropsychopharmacology 2009;34:390–8.

45. Burkhouse KL, Kujawa A, Klumpp H, et al. Neural correlates of explicit and implicit emotion processing in relation to treatment response in pediatric anxiety. J Child Psychol Psychiatry 2017;58:546–54.

46. Kujawa A, Swain JE, Hanna GL, et al. Prefrontal reactivity to social signals of threat as a predictor of treatment response in anxious youth. Neuropsychopharmacology 2016;41:1983–90.

47. Duong S, Chung K, Wigal SB. Metabolic, toxicological, and safety considerations for drugs used to treat ADHD. Expert Opin Drug Metab Toxicol 2012; 8:543–52.

48. Shaw P, Lerch J, Greenstein D, et al. Longitudinal mapping of cortical thickness and clinical outcome in children and adolescents with attention-deficit/hyperactivity disorder. Arch Gen Psychiatry 2006; 63:540–9.

49. Semrud-Clikeman M, Filipek PA, Biederman J, et al. Attention-deficit hyperactivity disorder: magnetic resonance imaging morphometric analysis of the corpus callosum. J Am Acad Child Adolesc Psychiatry 1994;33:875–81.

50. Filipek PA, Semrud-Clikeman M, Steingard RJ, et al. Volumetric MRI analysis comparing subjects having attention-deficit hyperactivity disorder with normal controls. Neurology 1997;48:589–601.

51. Mackie S, Shaw P, Lenroot R, et al. Cerebellar development and clinical outcome in attention deficit hyperactivity disorder. Am J Psychiatry 2007;164:647–55.

52. Moreno A, Duno L, Hoekzema E, et al. Striatal volume deficits in children with ADHD who present a poor response to methylphenidate. Eur Child Adolesc Psychiatry 2014;23:805–12.

53. Nakao T, Radua J, Rubia K, et al. Gray matter volume abnormalities in ADHD: voxel-based meta-analysis exploring the effects of age and stimulant medication. Am J Psychiatry 2011;168:1154–63.

54. Cho SC, Hwang JW, Kim BN, et al. The relationship between regional cerebral blood flow and response to methylphenidate in children with attention-deficit hyperactivity disorder: comparison between non-responders to methylphenidate and responders. J Psychiatr Res 2007;41:459–65.

55. Schweitzer JB, Lee DO, Hanford RB, et al. A positron emission tomography study of methylphenidate in adults with ADHD: alterations in resting blood flow and predicting treatment response. Neuropsychopharmacology 2003;28:967–73.

56. Amen DG, Hanks C, Prunella J. Predicting positive and negative treatment responses to stimulants with brain SPECT imaging. J Psychoactive Drugs 2008;40:131–8.

57. Cheon KA, Ryu YH, Kim JW, et al. The homozygosity for 10-repeat allele at dopamine transporter gene and dopamine transporter density in Korean children with attention deficit hyperactivity disorder: relating to treatment response to methylphenidate. Eur Neuropsychopharmacol 2005;15:95–101.

58. Ilgin N, Senol S, Gucuyener K, et al. Is increased D2 receptor availability associated with response to stimulant medication in ADHD. Dev Med Child Neurol 2001;43:755–60.

59. Krause J, la Fougere C, Krause KH, et al. Influence of striatal dopamine transporter availability on the response to methylphenidate in adult patients with ADHD. Eur Arch Psychiatry Clin Neurosci 2005; 255:428–31.

60. la Fougere C, Krause J, Krause KH, et al. Value of 99mTc-TRODAT-1 SPECT to predict clinical response to methylphenidate treatment in adults with attention deficit hyperactivity disorder. Nucl Med Commun 2006;27:733–7.

61. Hong SB, Harrison BJ, Fornito A, et al. Functional dysconnectivity of corticostriatal circuitry and differential response to methylphenidate in youth with attention-deficit/hyperactivity disorder. J Psychiatry Neurosci 2015;40:46–57.

62. Arns M. EEG-based personalized medicine in ADHD: individual alpha peak frequency as an endophenotype associated with nonresponse. J Neurotherapy 2012;16(2):123–41.

63. Li W, Li K, Guan P, et al. Volume alteration of hippocampal subfields in first-episode antipsychotic-naïve schizophrenia patients before and after acute antipsychotic treatment. Neuroimage Clin 2018;20:169–76.

64. Browning M, Kingslake J, Dourish CT, et al. Predicting treatment response to antidepressant medication using early changes in emotional processing. Eur Neuropsychopharmacol 2019;29:66–75.

65. Nord CL, Gray A, Charpentier CJ, et al. Unreliability of putative fMRI biomarkers during emotional face processing. Neuroimage 2017;156:119–27.

66. Deckert J, Erhardt A. Predicting treatment outcome for anxiety disorders with or without comorbid depression using clinical, imaging and (epi)genetic data. Curr Opin Psychiatry 2019;32:1–6.

67. Whitfield-Gabrieli S, Ghosh SS, Nieto-Castanon A, et al. Brain connectomics predict response to

treatment in social anxiety disorder. Mol Psychiatry 2016;21:680–5.

68. Kim JW, Sharma V, Ryan ND. Predicting methylphenidate response in ADHD using machine learning approaches. Int J Neuropsychopharmacol 2015; 18:pyv052.

69. Marquand AF, Rezek I, Buitelaar J, et al. Understanding heterogeneity in clinical cohorts using normative models: beyond case-control studies. Biol Psychiatry 2016;80:552–61.

70. Komulainen E, Heikkila R, Nummenmaa L, et al. Short-term escitalopram treatment normalizes aberrant self-referential processing in major depressive disorder. J Affect Disord 2018;236:222–9.

71. Klomp A, Caan MW, Denys D, et al. Feasibility of ASL-based phMRI with a single dose of oral citalopram for repeated assessment of serotonin function. Neuroimage 2012;63:1695–700.

72. Klomp A, van Wingen GA, de Ruiter MB, et al. Test-retest reliability of task-related pharmacological MRI with a single-dose oral citalopram challenge. Neuroimage 2013;75:108–16.

73. Schrantee A, Vaclavu L, Heijtel DF, et al. Dopaminergic system dysfunction in recreational dexamphetamine users. Neuropsychopharmacology 2015;40:1172–80.

74. Schrantee A, Solleveld MM, Schwantje H, et al. Dose-dependent effects of the selective serotonin reuptake inhibitor citalopram: a combined SPECT and phMRI study. J Psychopharmacol 2019;33: 660–9.

75. Klomp A, Tremoleda JL, Wylezinska M, et al. Lasting effects of chronic fluoxetine treatment on the late developing rat brain: age-dependent changes in the serotonergic neurotransmitter system assessed by pharmacological MRI. Neuroimage 2012;59: 218–26.

76. Schrantee A, Tamminga HG, Bouziane C, et al. Age-dependent effects of methylphenidate on the human dopaminergic system in young vs adult patients with attention-deficit/hyperactivity disorder: a randomized clinical trial. JAMA Psychiatry 2016;73: 955–62.

77. Henning A. Proton and multinuclear magnetic resonance spectroscopy in the human brain at ultra-high field strength: A review. Neuroimage 2018; 168:181–98.

Implementing MR Imaging into Clinical Routine Screening in Patients with Psychosis?

André Schmidt, PhD[a], Stefan Borgwardt, MD[a,b],*

KEYWORDS

• Psychoradiology • MR imaging • Psychosis

KEY POINTS

• MR imaging is a suitable instrument for the detection of incidental radiological findings in patients with early psychosis and guidance of subsequent treatment adjustments.
• Recent developments in data acquisition and quantitative analyses might further lead to objective diagnosis of organic psychosis.
• Besides identifying radiological abnormalities, MR imaging has emerged as a very powerful tool to map direct neurobiological processes associated with emerging psychosis.

INTRODUCTION

Engendered by the first modern MR imaging study[1] great enthusiasm and hope emerged that neuroimaging would help identifying the specific neurobiological pathology of psychosis. In contrast to the agnostic nature of the symptom-based clinical classification system about the underlying disease mechanisms,[2] neuroimaging is particularly promising because it is able to non-invasively capture pathophysiological abnormalities at its core, the brain. In particular, psychoradiology, an emerging subspecialty in the field of neuroradiology, mainly taking the advantage of MR imaging multimodal nature, is showing promise in its clinical application to the psychiatric illnesses.[3–6] The promise of MR imaging for the management of psychosis is to better understand the pathophysiology of psychotic symptoms at the very beginning of their development in order to apply early pathology tailored interventions. Interventions need directly target the pathophysiological processes causing psychosis in a manner that enduringly modifies its progression.[7] Discernible brain pathology associated with psychosis includes reductions in global and regional gray matter volume, ventricular enlargement, cerebral atrophy, and cavum septi pellucidi.[8,9] MR imaging provides a means of identifying such organic causes and could be used in the initial assessment of patients at early stages of psychosis.

Besides identifying radiological abnormalities, MR imaging has emerged as a very powerful tool to map direct neurobiological processes associated with emerging psychosis. Because it is not possible to predict clinical outcomes in subjects at increased risk of developing psychosis on the basis of the initial clinical baseline assessment,[10] there is a need for biomarkers such as brain markers that can help to improve the prediction of clinical outcomes in this group.[11] Numerous

Disclosure Statement: None.
^a Department of Psychiatry (UPK), University of Basel, Wilhelm Klein Strasse 27, Basel 4012, Switzerland;
^b Department of Psychiatry and Psychotherapy, University of Lübeck, Lübeck, Germany
* Corresponding author. Wilhelm Klein Strasse 27, Basel 4012, Switzerland.
E-mail address: s.borgwardt@unibas.ch

Neuroimag Clin N Am 30 (2020) 65–72
https://doi.org/10.1016/j.nic.2019.09.004
1052-5149/20/© 2019 The Authors. Published by Elsevier Inc. This is an open access article under the CC BY-NC-ND license (http://creativecommons.org/licenses/by-nc-nd/4.0/).

MR imaging studies have demonstrated that transition to full-blown psychosis is associated with structural and functional abnormalities in many different brain regions.[12–15] These findings gave rise to hope that routine MR imaging scanning could be used to stratify psychotic patients according to clinical outcome and subgroups of patients could then be offered different forms of treatment.[16–18]

As yet, however, MR imaging still has only a minor role in the clinical assessment of patients at early stages of psychosis and whether it should be implemented as routine screening instrument in psychotic patients has continued to generate debate.[19–21] In this article, we first outline evidence regarding the clinical utility of MR imaging to (1) detect neurological abnormalities and (2) predict clinical outcomes in patients at early stages of psychosis. It is then concluded whether it is reasonable to implement MR imaging as an initial clinical screening instrument now and present potential next developments.

MR IMAGING TO IDENTIFY RADIOLOGICAL ABNORMALITIES IN EARLY PSYCHOSIS

Although it is considered good practice to include a neuroimaging assessment in the initial clinical assessment of patients with psychosis,[22] this is not routinely carried out in all patients. Even though the proportion of patients with organic psychosis is small,[23] it is crucial to identify such radiological abnormalities as early as possible, as urgent treatment of the primary disease may be required.[24] Although it is widely acknowledged that MR imaging is suitable to identify organic causes of psychosis, it has been argued that scanning people with psychosis is too logistically difficult to be clinically worthwhile and might induce anxiety-related reactions.[25] From an economical point of view, a previous cost-effectiveness analysis found that MR imaging (and computed tomography) as part of the standard screening procedure is justifiable only if the prevalence rate for organic causes amenable to treatment is 1% and the time between presentation and assessment is less than 3 months.[19]

Radiological studies on the utility of MR imaging as clinical screening instrument provide inconsistent recommendations. A previous study reported radiological brain abnormalities in 22.2% of patients with first-episode psychosis (FEP) and in 50% of patients with chronic psychosis.[8] Seven percent and 19%, respectively, of patients in the 2 patient groups required routine referral based on this finding, whereas 2.0% and 1.1%, respectively, even required urgent referral. Given that MR imaging as part of the standard screening procedure is only justifiable if the prevalence rate for organic causes amenable to treatment is 1%,[19] this study[8] showed that even if only a small proportion of patients benefited directly from MR imaging scanning, it is economically worthwhile. In a more recent study, 11% of clinically relevant radiological abnormalities have been reported in patients with psychosis.[24] However, in contrast to Lubman and colleagues,[8] in this sample of 656 patients, none of the neuropathological findings observed have been interpreted as a possible substrate for organic psychosis. The investigators therefore concluded that radiological assessments of MR imaging scans should not be considered a necessary component of routine screening in psychotic patients, because the minimum economical rate of 1% is not met,[19] that is, at least 6 patients should have met criteria for organic psychosis in this sample.

A recently published article further contributed to this debate by first pointing out that the great majority of patients with psychosis were able to tolerate the scanning procedure very well, suggesting that an MR imaging assessment is practicable and logistically feasible in most patients with FEP, including patients in whom scanning is being done for clinical purposes.[20] Secondly, in accordance with other reports,[8,24,26,27] this study further observed that radiological abnormalities were relatively common in patients with FEP (6% of the research sample and 15% of the clinical sample), although they were also evident in healthy controls. None of the findings in patients with FEP entailed a change in clinical management. These results are comparable to a previous study in 37 people at clinical high risk for psychosis showing that radiological abnormalities are already present before the onset of the disorder.[9] Notably, the prevalence rates in high-risk subjects (35%) was similar to those in patients with FEP (40%).[9] They are unlikely to be related to antipsychotic medication, as most individuals at high risk and with FEP had never or only very briefly had been treated with antipsychotics.

Taken together, Falkenberg and colleagues[20] provide the most recent evidence for the clinical utility of MR imaging to detect gross brain abnormalities in patients with psychosis. The investigators concluded that MR imaging as part of the initial clinical assessment is feasible in most patients with FEP, even though most of them do not require a change in clinical management.[20] Nevertheless, aside from economic considerations,[19] the investigators[20] also emphasize that the consequences of failing to exclude such disorders in a young adult may be so grave that it is worth assessing everyone and suggest including MR imaging scans in the clinical assessment of all patients presenting with emerging psychosis.

MR IMAGING TO PREDICT CLINICAL OUTCOMES IN EARLY PSYCHOSIS

In addition to identifying organic psychosis, MR imaging is an indispensable tool to elucidate the neurobiological substrates that might underlie primary (or idiopathic) psychotic illness and in particular the transition to full-blown psychosis. Numerous imaging studies have demonstrated structural, functional, and chemical brain abnormalities[28–30] in clinical high-risk patients. Up to now, most studies used structural MR imaging to investigate alterations in regional gray matter volume in psychosis,[28] whereas some of them might predate the transition to psychosis.[31] Although such findings have significantly improved our understanding of the pathophysiological mechanisms underlying emerging psychosis, these group-level abnormalities do not capture individual deviations and therefore limit the prognostic accuracy of the data. Useful clinical predictions have to be made at the single-subject level. An established method for this purpose is the application of pattern recognition techniques, such as machine learning. These methods may promote an objective way to increase prognostic certainty to levels required for individualized prevention. Applying machine-learning approaches to neuroimaging data has the potential to revolutionize psychiatry by delivering prediction of individual patient outcome.[32] There has been an increase in the use and development of machine-learning techniques in clinical neuroscience[33] and in particular in the field of individualized early psychosis prediction.[34–40] Robust prediction models that are able to inform clinical outcomes in early phases of psychosis might be tremendously useful to stratify individual intervention scenarios. Using whole-brain gray matter volume, previous machine-learning studies demonstrated a more than 80% accuracy in predicting psychosis onset in clinical high-risk subjects.[40–42] Furthermore, it recently has been shown that the pattern of gray matter volume[43] can predict social functioning impairments in high-risk subjects with more than 75% accuracy. Notably, prognostic performance in the latter case could be significantly improved by combining information from clinical and MR imaging models.[43] Another study investigated whether cortical surface alterations analyzed by means of multivariate pattern recognition methods could enable the single-subject identification of functional outcomes in clinical high-risk individuals.[44]

Given that gray matter reductions seen in patients occur before the transition to psychosis, during the transition, or in the immediate postonset phase, morphometric methods such as the measurement of surface area or gyrification, are perhaps more sensitive to detect the pathophysiology in the prodromal phase.[45] Cortical surface-based pattern classification predicted good versus poor outcome status in clinical high-risk individuals with an accuracy of 82% as determined by nested leave-one-out-validation.[44] These results[43,44] are of high clinical relevance given that functioning may become worse even without transition to psychosis.[46]

More recent MR imaging studies revealed that brain abnormalities in psychosis are not solely attributable to changes in local regions and connections but rather emerge from changes in the topology of the network as a whole, the connectome of the brain.[47–53] Such network studies capture an important aspect of developmental maturation crucial for understanding the pathophysiology of psychotic disorders.[54,55] Previous studies reported reduced small-worldness of structural brain networks in patients with schizophrenia,[56–58] clinical high-risk subjects,[59] people at increased familial risk for schizophrenia,[60–62] and individuals with subclinical psychotic experiences,[63] characterized by increased segregation and reduced integration of anatomical covariance (see Refs.[54,64–67] for reviews of network analyses in psychosis). A recent study investigated whether transition to psychosis is associated with topological alterations in gyrification networks and whether this network information improves individual prediction of psychosis onset.[68] Gyrification is a compelling marker of early neurodevelopment and may be sensitive to detect the pathophysiology in the prodromal phase.[45] The findings of this cross-sectional MR imaging study showed that patients who develop psychosis reveal abnormalities in the gyrification-connectome and that topological measures of the gyrification-connectome predict the future outcome of transition with more than 80% accuracy.[68] This result highlights the potential of applying machine-learning techniques to brain connectome data to prognosticate clinical outcomes for psychosis in clinical high-risk individuals.[69]

IMPLEMENTING MR IMAGING AS ROUTINE SCREENING IN THE CLINIC: ARE WE THERE YET?

The potential of MR imaging for the detection of radiological abnormalities is undeniable and it has been shown that MR imaging as part of the clinical assessment is feasible in most patients with psychosis.[20] High-resolution MR imaging can now be acquired in a relatively short scanning time, which is particularly useful in patients who may be acutely unwell. Although abnormalities that could account for a psychosis are rare, the impact of missing them is so tremendous that it is well justified to assess everyone with current acquisition protocols. However, identification of actionable brain pathology is so insufficient that it is not a good allocation of health care resources in a resource limited environment. Implementing MR imaging as a standard screening tool would also help to collect more data and thereby enhance the possibility to identify radiological abnormalities other than the already familiar ones. Diagnoses of organic psychosis might be further improved with the development of new diagnostic assessments. For instance, T2 or fluid-attenuated inversion recovery hyperintensities may help to detect psychotic patients with anti-NMDAR encephalitis.[70] Furthermore, although radiological examinations are still based on visual inspection, the development of quantitative analytical approaches (such as machine learning) might help to make objective diagnoses of organic psychosis in the near future.

High-resolution MR imaging combined with sophisticated quantitative analyses may not only improve the detection of organic causes but also the prediction of clinical outcomes (eg, transition, functioning) in high-risk subjects. Although previous results from machine-learning studies designed to predict clinical outcomes in high-risk subjects are promising,[40–43,68] major hurdles lie ahead before MR imaging is ready to be implemented in the clinic for prognostic assessments. The first issue is that most studies are clearly underpowered. To exploit the entire potential of MR imaging and to ultimately evaluate its prognostic utility for psychiatric services, we need quantitative results from large patient samples using predefined research protocols. Currently ongoing multicenter studies, such as PRONIA (Personalized Prognostic Tools for Early Psychosis Management), PSYSCAN (Translating Neuroimaging Findings From Research Into Clinical Practice), and NAPLS (North American Prodrome Longitudinal Study), will be able to address this issue by delivering large samples. Once outcomes are defined using well-established and clinically meaningful criteria, outcome-specific predictors need to be selected[71] by considering, for instance, evidence from systematic reviews or meta-analysis.[72] Given that psychosis is best understood in terms of brain network dysfunction rather than

by abnormalities in isolated brain regions,[47–53] brain network markers might be particularly promising to determine staging of psychosis.[13,73,74] A prognostic model also can consist of predictors from the same imaging modality (eg, volume, surface, or gyrification data) or across different modalities (eg, structural and functional MR imaging data). In any case, it is critical to consider the incidence of the outcome, that is, that the event per variable ratio is at least 10.[75] Integrating MR imaging data with nonimaging measures that have independently been linked with altered outcomes in psychosis (eg, polygenic risk score, inflammatory markers) may also enhance predictive power, although it has yet to be tested.[16] Similarly, it is also possible to combine MR imaging data with clinical data, as recently demonstrated,[43] given that biological assays such as MR imaging will unlikely replace clinical assessments but might help to supplement them.[76] The simplest approach for data fusion is to concatenate all data into the same model.[69] It is also possible to combine the prognostic performance across separate models (eg, clinical and MR imaging model) by using ensemble learning strategies[77] or a multistage sequential testing approach.[11,78] After feature selection and data preparation (including proper handling of missing data),[75] prognostic models can be developed.[72] A critical step during model development is to estimate the model's performance using internal validation methods to adjust for optimism.[72] Internal validation is performed on the development data set by fitting the model in a training data set and then assessing performance in a test data set of unseen cases from the same population.[72] Frequent internal validation methods are k-fold cross-validation and bootstrapping.[75] To address heterogeneity across patients is then essential to test the generalizability of the developed model on individuals outside the development set.[79] The less the validation differs from the development sample, the stronger the test of generalizability of the model.[80] To our knowledge, no prognostic MR imaging model in psychotic patients has been externally validated up to now. Once these models have been validated on external (new) data sets in prospective patient studies, which is most challenging, these technologies need to be implemented into real-world clinical routine. Model impact studies with a comparative design are needed to test whether prediction models change individuals' or health care professionals' behavior or clinical decision making.[81,82] Easy-to-use Web-based interfaces that can automatically give predictions for individual patients can certainly improve implementation processes.[83] Such online calculators using clinical and demographic data have been provided for the prediction of psychosis onset in clinical high-risk individuals[84] and is being implemented in a national health system.[85]

SUMMARY

In conclusion, this article first outlines the clinical utility of MR imaging to identify radiological abnormalities in psychotic patients and suggests that an initial MR imaging assessment is indicated in early stages of the disorder. Recent developments in data acquisition and quantitative analyses might further lead to objective diagnosis of organic psychosis. Although first evidence is promising,[40–44,68] we further show that MR imaging-based prognostic models for individuals at early stages of psychosis are not yet ready to be implemented as clinical baseline assessment. Further progress requires the collection of large samples, selection of standardized outcome-specific predictors, a methodologically sound development of prognostic models, and their validation in large independent samples. The field is armed to tackle these challenges and to exploit the entire potential of MR imaging for clinical decision making in early detection and intervention services.

REFERENCES

1. Johnstone EC, Crow TJ, Frith CD, et al. Cerebral ventricular size and cognitive impairment in chronic schizophrenia. Lancet 1976;2(7992):924–6.
2. Stephan KE, Bach DR, Fletcher PC, et al. Charting the landscape of priority problems in psychiatry, part 1: classification and diagnosis. Lancet Psychiatry 2016;3(1):77–83.
3. Danhong W, Meiling L, Meiyun W, et al. Individual-specific functional connectivity markers track dimensional and categorical features of psychotic illness. Mol Psychiatry 2018. [Epub ahead of print].
4. Huang X, Gong Q, Sweeney JA, et al. Progress in psychoradiology, the clinical application of psychiatric neuroimaging. Br J Radiol 2019;92(1101):20181000.
5. Port JD. Diagnosis of attention deficit hyperactivity disorder by using MR imaging and radiomics: a potential tool for clinicians. Radiology 2018;287:631–2.
6. Sun H, Chen Y, Huang Q, et al. Psychoradiologic utility of MR imaging for diagnosis of attention deficit hyperactivity disorder: a radiomics analysis. Radiology 2018;287(2):620–30.
7. Millan MJ, Andrieux A, Bartzokis G, et al. Altering the course of schizophrenia: progress and perspectives. Nat Rev Drug Discov 2016;15(7):485–515.
8. Lubman DI, Velakoulis D, McGorry PD, et al. Incidental radiological findings on brain magnetic resonance imaging in first-episode psychosis and chronic schizophrenia. Acta Psychiatr Scand 2002;106(5):331–6.
9. Borgwardt SJ, Radue EW, Götz K, et al. Radiological findings in individuals at high risk of psychosis. J Neurol Neurosurg Psychiatry 2006;77(2):229–33.
10. Fusar-Poli P, Cappucciati M, Rutigliano G, et al. At risk or not at risk? A meta-analysis of the prognostic accuracy of psychometric interviews for psychosis prediction. World Psychiatry 2015;14(3):322–32.
11. Schmidt A, Cappucciati M, Radua J, et al. Improving prognostic accuracy in subjects at clinical high risk for psychosis: systematic review of predictive models and meta-analytical sequential testing simulation. Schizophr Bull 2016;43(2):375–88.
12. Smieskova R, Fusar-Poli P, Allen P, et al. Neuroimaging predictors of transition to psychosis–a systematic review and meta-analysis. Neurosci Biobehav Rev 2010;34(8):1207–22.
13. Schmidt A, Diwadkar VA, Smieskova R, et al. Approaching a network connectivity-driven classification of the psychosis continuum: a selective review and suggestions for future research. Front Hum Neurosci 2014;8:1047.
14. Pettersson-Yeo W, Allen P, Benetti S, et al. Dysconnectivity in schizophrenia: where are we now? Neurosci Biobehav Rev 2011;35(5):1110–24.
15. Bois C, Whalley HC, McIntosh AM, et al. Structural magnetic resonance imaging markers of susceptibility and transition to schizophrenia: a review of familial and clinical high risk population studies. J Psychopharmacol 2015;29(2):144–54.
16. McGuire P, Dazzan P. Does neuroimaging have a role in predicting outcomes in psychosis? World Psychiatry 2017;16(2):209–10.
17. McGuire P, Sato JR, Mechelli A, et al. Can neuroimaging be used to predict the onset of psychosis? Lancet Psychiatry 2015;2(12):1117–22.
18. Gifford G, Crossley N, Fusar-Poli P, et al. Using neuroimaging to help predict the onset of psychosis. Neuroimage 2017;145(Pt B):209–17.
19. Albon E, Tsourapas A, Frew E, et al. Structural neuroimaging in psychosis: a systematic review and economic evaluation. Health Technol Assess 2008;12(18):iii–iv, ix–163.
20. Falkenberg I, Benetti S, Raffin M, et al. Clinical utility of magnetic resonance imaging in first-episode psychosis. Br J Psychiatry 2017;211(4):231–7.
21. Borgwardt S, Schmidt A. Is neuroimaging clinically useful in subjects at high risk for psychosis? World Psychiatry 2016;15(2):178–9.
22. Gaebel W, Falkai P, Weinmann S, et al. Praxisleitlinien in Psychiatrie und Psychotherapie, Band 1, Behandlungsleitlinie Schizophrenie. Deutsche Gesellschaft

für Psychiatrie, Psychotherapie und Nervenheilkunde (DGPPN), 2006.

23. Falkai P. Differential diagnosis in acute psychotic episode. Int Clin Psychopharmacol 1996;11(Suppl 2):13–7.

24. Sommer IE, de Kort GA, Meijering AL, et al. How frequent are radiological abnormalities in patients with psychosis? A review of 1379 MRI scans. Schizophr Bull 2013;39(4):815–9.

25. Khandanpour N, Hoggard N, Connolly DJ. The role of MRI and CT of the brain in first episodes of psychosis. Clin Radiol 2013;68(3):245–50.

26. Lieberman J, Bogerts B, Degreef G, et al. Qualitative assessment of brain morphology in acute and chronic schizophrenia. Am J Psychiatry 1992; 149(6):784–94.

27. Lawrie SM, Abukmeil SS, Chiswick A, et al. Qualitative cerebral morphology in schizophrenia: a magnetic resonance imaging study and systematic literature review. Schizophr Res 1997;25(2): 155–66.

28. Fusar-Poli P, Radua J, McGuire P, et al. Neuroanatomical maps of psychosis onset: voxel-wise meta-analysis of antipsychotic-naive VBM studies. Schizophr Bull 2012;38(6):1297–307.

29. Radua J, Schmidt A, Borgwardt S, et al. Ventral striatal activation during reward processing in psychosis: a neurofunctional meta-analysis. JAMA Psychiatry 2015;72(12):1243–51.

30. Howes OD, Bose SK, Turkheimer F, et al. Dopamine synthesis capacity before onset of psychosis: a prospective [18F]-DOPA PET imaging study. Am J Psychiatry 2011;168(12):1311–7.

31. Mechelli A, Riecher-Rössler A, Meisenzahl EM, et al. Neuroanatomical abnormalities that predate the onset of psychosis: a multicenter study. Arch Gen Psychiatry 2011;68(5):489–95.

32. Darcy AM, Louie AK, Roberts LW. Machine learning and the profession of medicine. JAMA 2016;315(6): 551–2.

33. Pereira F, Mitchell T, Botvinick M. Machine learning classifiers and fMRI: a tutorial overview. Neuroimage 2009;45(1 Suppl):S199–209.

34. Salvador R, Radua J, Canales-Rodríguez EJ, et al. Evaluation of machine learning algorithms and structural features for optimal MRI-based diagnostic prediction in psychosis. PLoS One 2017; 12(4):e0175683.

35. Schreiner M, Forsyth JK, Karlsgodt KH, et al. Intrinsic connectivity network-based classification and detection of psychotic symptoms in youth with 22q11.2 deletions. Cereb Cortex 2017;27(6): 3294–306.

36. Mechelli A, Lin A, Wood S, et al. Using clinical information to make individualized prognostic predictions in people at ultra high risk for psychosis. Schizophr Res 2017;184:32–8.

37. de Wit S, Ziermans TB, Nieuwenhuis M, et al. Individual prediction of long-term outcome in adolescents at ultra-high risk for psychosis: applying machine learning techniques to brain imaging data. Hum Brain Mapp 2017;38(2):704–14.

38. Young J, Kempton MJ, McGuire P. Using machine learning to predict outcomes in psychosis. Lancet Psychiatry 2016;3(10):908–9.

39. Bendfeldt K, Smieskova R, Koutsouleris N, et al. Classifying individuals at high-risk for psychosis based on functional brain activity during working memory processing. Neuroimage Clin 2015;9: 555–63.

40. Koutsouleris N, Riecher-Rössler A, Meisenzahl EM, et al. Detecting the psychosis prodrome across high-risk populations using neuroanatomical biomarkers. Schizophr Bull 2015;41(2):471–82.

41. Koutsouleris N, Meisenzahl EM, Davatzikos C, et al. Use of neuroanatomical pattern classification to identify subjects in at-risk mental states of psychosis and predict disease transition. Arch Gen Psychiatry 2009;66(7):700–12.

42. Koutsouleris N, Borgwardt S, Meisenzahl EM, et al. Disease prediction in the at-risk mental state for psychosis using neuroanatomical biomarkers: results from the FePsy study. Schizophr Bull 2012;38(6): 1234–46.

43. Koutsouleris N, Kambeitz-Ilankovic L, Ruhrmann S, et al. Prediction models of functional outcomes for individuals in the clinical high-risk state for psychosis or with recent-onset depression: a multimodal, multisite machine learning analysis. JAMA Psychiatry 2018;75(11):1156–72.

44. Kambeitz-Ilankovic L, Meisenzahl EM, Cabral C, et al. Prediction of outcome in the psychosis prodrome using neuroanatomical pattern classification. Schizophr Res 2016;173(3):159–65.

45. Palaniyappan L. Progressive cortical reorganisation: a framework for investigating structural changes in schizophrenia. Neurosci Biobehav Rev 2017;79: 1–13.

46. Addington J, Cornblatt BA, Cadenhead KS, et al. At clinical high risk for psychosis: outcome for non-converters. Am J Psychiatry 2011;168(8):800–5.

47. van den Heuvel MP, Mandl RC, Stam CJ, et al. Aberrant frontal and temporal complex network structure in schizophrenia: a graph theoretical analysis. J Neurosci 2010;30(47):15915–26.

48. Filippi M, van den Heuvel MP, Fornito A, et al. Assessment of system dysfunction in the brain through MRI-based connectomics. Lancet Neurol 2013;12(12):1189–99.

49. Fornito A, Zalesky A, Breakspear M. The connectomics of brain disorders. Nat Rev Neurosci 2015; 16(3):159–72.

50. Crossley NA, Mechelli A, Scott J, et al. The hubs of the human connectome are generally implicated in

the anatomy of brain disorders. Brain 2014;137(Pt 8):2382–95.

51. Fornito A, Bullmore ET, Zalesky A. Opportunities and challenges for psychiatry in the connectomic era. Biol Psychiatry Cogn Neurosci Neuroimaging 2017; 2:9–19.

52. Crossley NA, Mechelli A, Ginestet C, et al. Altered hub functioning and compensatory activations in the connectome: a meta-analysis of functional neuroimaging studies in schizophrenia. Schizophr Bull 2016;42(2):434–42.

53. Rubinov M, Bullmore E. Fledgling pathoconnectomics of psychiatric disorders. Trends Cogn Sci 2013; 17(12):641–7.

54. Alexander-Bloch A, Giedd JN, Bullmore E. Imaging structural co-variance between human brain regions. Nat Rev Neurosci 2013;14(5):322–36.

55. Evans AC. Networks of anatomical covariance. Neuroimage 2013;80:489–504.

56. Bassett DS, Bullmore E, Verchinski BA, et al. Hierarchical organization of human cortical networks in health and schizophrenia. J Neurosci 2008;28(37): 9239–48.

57. Zhang Y, Lin L, Lin CP, et al. Abnormal topological organization of structural brain networks in schizophrenia. Schizophr Res 2012;141(2–3):109–18.

58. van den Heuvel MP, Sporns O, Collin G, et al. Abnormal rich club organization and functional brain dynamics in schizophrenia. JAMA Psychiatry 2013; 70(8):783–92.

59. Schmidt A, Crossley NA, Harrisberger F, et al. Structural network disorganization in subjects at clinical high risk for psychosis. Schizophr Bull 2016;43(3): 583–91.

60. Tijms BM, Sprooten E, Job D, et al. Grey matter networks in people at increased familial risk for schizophrenia. Schizophr Res 2015;168(1–2):1–8.

61. Shi F, Yap PT, Gao W, et al. Altered structural connectivity in neonates at genetic risk for schizophrenia: a combined study using morphological and white matter networks. Neuroimage 2012; 62(3):1622–33.

62. Yan H, Tian L, Wang Q, et al. Compromised small-world efficiency of structural brain networks in schizophrenic patients and their unaffected parents. Neurosci Bull 2015;31(3):275–87.

63. Drakesmith M, Caeyenberghs K, Dutt A, et al. Schizophrenia-like topological changes in the structural connectome of individuals with subclinical psychotic experiences. Hum Brain Mapp 2015;36(7): 2629–43.

64. Fornito A, Zalesky A, Pantelis C, et al. Schizophrenia, neuroimaging and connectomics. Neuroimage 2012;62(4):2296–314.

65. Fornito A, Bullmore ET. Reconciling abnormalities of brain network structure and function in schizophrenia. Curr Opin Neurobiol 2015;30:44–50.

66. van den Heuvel MP, Fornito A. Brain networks in schizophrenia. Neuropsychol Rev 2014;24(1): 32–48.

67. Rubinov M, Bullmore E. Schizophrenia and abnormal brain network hubs. Dialogues Clin Neurosci 2013;15(3):339–49.

68. Das T, Borgwardt S, Hauke DJ, et al. Disorganized gyrification network properties during the transition to psychosis. JAMA Psychiatry 2018;75(6):613–22.

69. Walter M, Alizadeh S, Jamalabadi H, et al. Translational machine learning for psychiatric neuroimaging. Prog Neuropsychopharmacol Biol Psychiatry 2019;91:113–21.

70. Dalmau J, Lancaster E, Martinez-Hernandez E, et al. Clinical experience and laboratory investigations in patients with anti-NMDAR encephalitis. Lancet Neurol 2011;10(1):63–74.

71. Moons KG, Altman DG, Vergouwe Y, et al. Prognosis and prognostic research: application and impact of prognostic models in clinical practice. BMJ 2009; 338:b606.

72. Fusar-Poli P, Hijazi Z, Stahl D, et al. The science of prognosis in psychiatry: a review. JAMA Psychiatry 2018;75(12):1289–97.

73. Deco G, Kringelbach ML. Great expectations: using whole-brain computational connectomics for understanding neuropsychiatric disorders. Neuron 2014; 84(5):892–905.

74. Castellanos FX, Di Martino A, Craddock RC, et al. Clinical applications of the functional connectome. Neuroimage 2013;80:527–40.

75. Studerus E, Ramyead A, Riecher-Rössler A. Prediction of transition to psychosis in patients with a clinical high risk for psychosis: a systematic review of methodology and reporting. Psychol Med 2017; 47(7):1163–78.

76. Kapur S, Phillips AG, Insel TR. Why has it taken so long for biological psychiatry to develop clinical tests and what to do about it? Mol Psychiatry 2012;17(12):1174–9.

77. Polikar R. Ensemble based systems in decision making. IEEE Circuits and Systems Magazine 2006;6(3):21–45.

78. Clark SR, Schubert KO, Baune BT. Towards indicated prevention of psychosis: using probabilistic assessments of transition risk in psychosis prodrome. J Neural Transm (Vienna) 2015;122(1): 155–69.

79. Justice AC, Covinsky KE, Berlin JA. Assessing the generalizability of prognostic information. Ann Intern Med 1999;130(6):515–24.

80. Moons KG, Kengne AP, Grobbee DE, et al. Risk prediction models: II. External validation, model updating, and impact assessment. Heart 2012;98(9): 691–8.

81. Reilly BM, Evans AT. Translating clinical research into clinical practice: impact of using prediction

rules to make decisions. Ann Intern Med 2006; 144(3):201–9.

82. Wallace E, Smith SM, Perera-Salazar R, et al. Framework for the impact analysis and implementation of Clinical Prediction Rules (CPRs). BMC Med Inform Decis Mak 2011;11:62.

83. Chekroud AM, Koutsouleris N. The perilous path from publication to practice. Mol Psychiatry 2018; 23(1):24–5.

84. Cannon TD, Yu C, Addington J, et al. An individualized risk calculator for research in prodromal psychosis. Am J Psychiatry 2016;173(10): 980–8.

85. Fusar-Poli P, Werbeloff N, Rutigliano G, et al. Transdiagnostic risk calculator for the automatic detection of individuals at risk and the prediction of psychosis: second replication in an independent national health service trust. Schizophr Bull 2018;45(3):562–70.

Neuroimaging in Schizophrenia

Matcheri S. Keshavan, MD[a,*], Guusje Collin, PhD[b,c], Synthia Guimond, PhD[d], Sinead Kelly, PhD[a], Konasale M. Prasad, MD[e,f,g], Paulo Lizano, MD, PhD[a]

KEYWORDS

- Schizophrenia • Magnetic resonance imaging • Psychoradiology • Structural • Functional
- Spectroscopy • Diffusion • Diagnosis

KEY POINTS

- Neuroimaging studies have shown substantive evidence of brain structural, functional, and neurochemical alterations in schizophrenia, consistent with the neurodevelopmental and neurodegenerative models of this illness.
- The observed alterations are not regionally specific, but are more pronounced in the association cortex (prefrontal, parietal, and temporal) and subcortical (limbic, striatal) brain regions.
- Individually observed abnormalities across psychiatric disorders are not sufficiently specific yet to be of diagnostic value.
- Future research should pay attention to multivariate machine learning approaches, multisite consortia for large sample sizes, prospective studies and novel approaches to address emerging genetic, synaptic, and neurochemical models of schizophrenia pathophysiology.

INTRODUCTION

Psychotic disorders are mental illnesses characterized by difficulties in reality testing.[1] Schizophrenia is a severe and chronic psychotic disorder with a lifetime prevalence of about 1%. Onset is typically in adolescence or early adulthood; characteristic symptoms include abnormally held beliefs (delusions), altered perceptions (hallucinations), disordered thinking, disorganized behavior (collectively positive symptoms) and deficits in motivation, affect, and socialization (negative symptoms). Diagnosis of schizophrenia, by the *Diagnostic and Statistical Manual of Mental Disorders*, 5th edition,[2] requires the presence of at least 2 of these symptoms, along with a decline in functioning, lasting at least 6 months, and ensuring that these symptoms cannot be better explained by another medical disease, substance use or another psychiatric disorder. Impairments in cognition in recent years have emerged as central features underlying the disability in schizophrenia.[3]

WHAT IS CURRENTLY KNOWN ABOUT THE NEUROBIOLOGY OF SCHIZOPHRENIA

Schizophrenia has been increasingly viewed as a disorder of brain development.[4–6] Abnormalities in early brain development, around or before birth,

Disclosure Statement: None.
[a] Beth Israel Deaconess Medical Center, Harvard Medical School, 75 Fenwood Road, Boston, MA 02115, USA; [b] McGovern Institute for Brain Research, Massachusetts Institute of Technology, 43 Vassar St, Cambridge, MA 02139, USA; [c] University Medical Center Utrecht Brain Center, Heidelberglaan 100, Postbus 85500, 3508 GA, Utrecht, the Netherlands; [d] Department of Psychiatry, The Royal's Institute of Mental Health Research, University of Ottawa, 1145 Carling Avenue, Ottawa, ON K1Z 7K4, Canada; [e] University of Pittsburgh School of Medicine, Suite 279, 3811 O'Hara St, Pittsburgh, PA 15213, USA; [f] Swanson School of Engineering, University of Pittsburgh, Pittsburgh, PA, USA; [g] Veterans Affairs Pittsburgh Healthcare System, Pittsburgh, PA, USA
* Corresponding author. BIDMC-Mass. Mental Health Center, 75 Fenwood Road, Boston, MA 02115.
E-mail address: keshavanms@gmail.com

as well as late developmental derailments around or before the onset of psychosis have been proposed. It has been suggested that programmed pruning during adolescence may be excessive leading to the emergence of the illness, consistent with observed reductions in cortical dendrite density.[7] Postillness onset degenerative processes may also be involved.[8] Neuroimaging studies have the potential to examine predictions generated by these seemingly contrasting models. We review the current status of the burgeoning imaging literature across several imaging modalities (structural, functional, and neurochemical) that has accumulated during recent years to illuminate the putative causal mechanisms and may help to improve our approaches to diagnosis, outcome prediction, and treatment selection.

IMAGING BRAIN STRUCTURE AND WHITE MATTER CONNECTIONS

Brain structural abnormalities are widely reported in schizophrenia with large-scale meta-analyses detecting a smaller hippocampal volume in patients compared with controls, followed by smaller amygdala, thalamus, nucleus accumbens, and intracranial volumes, as well as larger pallidum and lateral ventricle volumes.[9] Individuals with schizophrenia also have widespread cortical thinning and a smaller cortical surface area, with the greatest effects observed in frontal and temporal lobe regions.[10] Differences in cortical thickness are found to be more regionally specific, whereas cortical surface area effects are more global.[10] Cortical thickness decreases are also more pronounced in individuals receiving antipsychotic medication and negatively correlate with medication dose, symptom severity, and duration of illness.[10] Advances in neuroimaging methods have led to a dysconnectivity hypothesis of schizophrenia, whereby the disorder may involve abnormal or inefficient communication between functional brain regions[11] contributed by abnormalities in the underlying white matter connections. Notably psychoradiology, a subspecialty of radiology pioneered by Gong and his colleagues (https://radiopaedia.org/articles/psychoradiology),[12–14] is showing promise in guiding clinical management of psychiatric disorders.[13,15]

As one of most important tools for psychoradiology, diffusion tensor imaging allows for the in vivo study of white matter microstructure. Diffusion tensor imaging studies of schizophrenia typically report lower fractional anisotropy (FA; a value ranging from 0 to 1 that reflects the degree of freedom for water molecules to diffuse in all directions) in patients compared with controls, typically in the fiber tracts connecting prefrontal and temporal lobes.[16,17] However, recent meta-analytic findings suggest that FA decreases are more widespread in schizophrenia, affecting almost all major white matter regions with largest effects observed for cortical–thalamic and interhemispheric tracts, including the corona radiata and corpus callosum.[5]

Although structural and diffusion imaging studies have shed light on the underlying neurobiology of schizophrenia,[14,18–20] the majority of these studies examine chronic patients and individuals taking antipsychotic medications,[21] with the exception of the milestone discovery of the brain structural deficit and symptom association in first-episode patients, as reported by Lui and colleagues.[19] Therefore, it is difficult to identify the timing of brain changes and the effects of medication exposure. Additional studies examining populations before illness onset, as well as longitudinal studies throughout the course of the illness, are warranted. Furthermore, advanced neuroimaging methodologies such as diffusion tensor imaging are limited in their ability to identify the type of underlying pathology. For example, lower FA may reflect abnormal fiber coherence or packing, or alterations of axonal integrity and/or myelination. Future studies using more advanced diffusion MR imaging methods, such as free water imaging, may offer increased sensitivity to subtle brain abnormalities, as well as improved specificity to pathologies such as neuroinflammation or demyelination.[22]

IMAGING BRAIN FUNCTION AND PERFUSION

It is well-established that brain function parallels changes in brain structure, which can be assessed using functional neuroimaging studies. Because cerebral blood flow is tightly coupled to brain metabolism, early neuroimaging studies measured cerebral blood flow using [133]Xenon inhalation[23] or various radiotracers in single photon emission computed tomography (SPECT),[24] whereas PET techniques were used to measure metabolism (^{11}C-glucose and fluorine-18 fluorodeoxyglucose tracers)[25] and blood flow (oxygen-15 tracer).[26] Advances in neuroscientific methods which improved on cost, time, and patient burden have favored the use of 2 in vivo techniques: blood oxygenation level-dependent functional MR imaging (fMR imaging) and arterial spin labeled (ASL) perfusion MR imaging. These techniques provide robust, balanced (spatial and temporal resolution), and clinically relevant correlates of neural activity and microvascular function in schizophrenia. Whereas fMR imaging can robustly measure neuronal activity indirectly through changes in blood flow and oxygen metabolism,[27] ASL measures cerebral blood flow directly by inverting the magnetization of the arterial blood water using radiofrequency pulses to create an endogenous diffusible tracer.[28] Unlike PET or SPECT, fMR imaging and ASL are noninvasive and do not require ionizing radiation, relying rather on the magnetic properties of the brain's natural elements.

Alterations in brain metabolism and blood flow have been demonstrated in a meta-analysis of [133]xenon, SPECT and PET studies, where Hill and colleagues[29] (2004) identified evidence for a resting hypofrontality with small-to-medium effect sizes in patients with schizophrenia, with chronic patients showing the largest effects. Hill and colleagues[29] (2004) also demonstrated evidence for task-activated hypofrontality, with medium effect size differences in executive, vigilance, and memory tasks, and showed that poorer performance was associated with greater hypofrontality. In a meta-analysis of PET and fMR imaging studies of working memory in schizophrenia, Glahn and colleagues[30] (2005) found that, in addition to hypofrontality, there is also increased activation in the anterior cingulate and left frontal pole regions. Abnormal resting state brain activity has also been reported in a meta-analysis of studies using PET, fMR imaging, and ASL and the authors identified hypoactivation in the ventromedial prefrontal cortex, left hippocampus, posterior cingulate cortex, precuneus, and hyperactivation in the bilateral lingual gyrus of schizophrenic patients compared with controls.[31] Last, in a systematic review of ASL imaging in schizophrenia, the authors identified convergent decreases in cerebral blood flow in the frontal lobe, left middle frontal gyrus, inferior frontal gyrus, lingual gyrus, cuneus, middle occipital gyrus, fusiform gyrus, anterior cingulate, and parietal lobe, with the putamen as the only region showing increased cerebral blood flow in schizophrenia.[32] The same study also found inconsistent results for the middle temporal, parahippocampal, precuneus, and thalamic regions.[32] Taken together, functional imaging studies point toward altered metabolic or hemodynamic activity in frontal, cingulate, parietal, and occipital brain regions with a few areas of hyperactivity, such as the putamen and sensorimotor regions, but more work is needed to determine the clinical implications of these observations.

IMAGING BRAIN CHEMISTRY

PET, SPECT, and magnetic resonance spectroscopy (MRS) have been extensively used to investigate chemical changes in the brain. PET imaging studies have examined the receptors of interest to schizophrenia, primarily dopamine, serotonin, gamma aminobutyric acid (GABA), and glutamate. PET studies have provided direct evidence of D_2/D_3 receptors as the primary site of action of most antipsychotic drugs.[33] Dopamine D_2 receptor density and occupancy of D_2 receptors by dopamine has been shown to be increased in patients with schizophrenia[34] along with increased dopamine transmission.[35] Although increased in patients, D_2 receptor density is not a consistent marker discriminating patients with schizophrenia and controls.[36] Striatal dopamine transporter availability is also not different between healthy controls and medication-naïve patients with schizophrenia.[37] By contrast, several studies have shown that patients with schizophrenia show a modest but significant increase in dopamine synthesis capacity compared with controls.[38]

Examinations of other neurotransmitter receptors have provided important leads in understanding the pathophysiology of schizophrenia. A meta-analysis of PET studies reported reduced serotonin (5-HT)$_1$ receptors in the midbrain and pons, and reduced 5-HT$_2$ receptors in the neocortex with no changes in serotonin transporter relative to controls.[39] The glutamate system has also been investigated using PET and proton MRS (^{1}H MRS). A review of these studies suggested hypofunction of N-methyl-D-aspartate receptors in schizophrenia.[40] A meta-analysis of ^{1}H MRS GABA studies did not show significant differences in GABA levels between patients and controls.[41] Even PET/SPECT studies do not show replicable differences,[42] although findings that GABA dynamics may be different in medicated and nonmedicated patients[43] could contribute to the inconsistent results observed in case control studies. Similarly, meta-analyses of ^{1}H MRS studies on glutamate alterations in schizophrenia have resulted in inconsistent results. One meta-analysis reported decreased glutamate and increased glutamine in the medial frontal region in patients with schizophrenia.[44] A later meta-analysis reported elevation of glutamate in basal ganglia, glutamine in the thalamus, and glutamate plus glutamine in the thalamus and medial temporal lobe,[45] but no specific brain region showing decreased glutamate levels in schizophrenia.

Overall, these findings suggest that the evidence for dopamine dysfunction is more replicable than that for other neurotransmitter systems. However, these neurotransmitters do not work in isolation, and changes in these systems may vary with the course of the illness. For example, feedback neural circuitry involving glutamate, GABA, and dopamine is essential for regulating dopamine transmission in the striatum. Furthermore, GABA (an inhibitory neurotransmitter) modulates dopamine release in the frontal cortex and striatum is regulated by glutamate (an excitatory neurotransmitter) through N-methyl-D-aspartate receptors. A hypoglutamatergic state can lead to reduced inhibition of dopamine, which in turn could lead to increased dopamine secretion/synthesis. Thus, the excitation/inhibition balance between GABA and glutamate is proposed to be central to the regulation of dopamine.

MRS studies have examined the brain biology of schizophrenia apart from neurotransmitter alterations. N-Acetyl aspartate, a marker of neuronal viability, has been found to be reduced in different regions of the brain, including the prefrontal cortex, temporal lobe and the thalamus. Phosphorus MRS (^{31}P MRS) studies, which assess differences in membrane expansion/contraction of cellular components by quantifying precursors (phosphomonoesters) and catabolites (phosphodiesters) of membrane phospholipids, have demonstrated regionally specific imbalances in membrane phospholipid metabolism related to neuropil in patients with schizophrenia compared with controls reflecting neuropil contraction. In addition, decreased phosphomonoester levels in frontal regions, and elevated phosphodiester levels in temporal regions provide evidence of decreased synthesis and increased degradation of neuropil membrane, respectively.[46] Another method called phosphorus magnetization transfer MRS has been applied to examine cerebral bioenergetics. Using this method, reduced creatine kinase forward reaction constant has been observed in the frontal lobes of patients with schizophrenia, suggesting an altered regeneration of adenosine triphosphate, a high-energy metabolite.[47]

DIAGNOSTIC VALUE OF IMAGING IN SCHIZOPHRENIA

The diagnosis of schizophrenia currently primarily depends on clinical assessments based on psychiatric history and mental status examination. Laboratory tests and imaging procedures have so far been used mainly to rule out disorders that cause secondary psychosis such as medical illnesses and substance abuse. Lubman and colleagues[48] (2002) observed that nearly 30% of all brain scans of patients with schizophrenia are reported as abnormal by radiologists, but the majority were seen as not clinically significant. Only a small proportion (4/340) of scan findings lead to the discovery of a previously unsuspected pathology. This suggests that the routine use of brain scans to rule out neuropathology in psychotic patients may not be cost effective.[49]

Current classification systems such as the *Diagnostic and Statistical Manual of Mental Disorders* and the International Classification of Diseases do not include any biomarkers as part of the diagnostic schemes for psychotic disorders. However, there has been an increasing interest in developing reliable objective biomarkers including those involving neuroimaging data to rule in a diagnosis by supplementing clinical approaches to diagnosis. The literature has showed the potential of neuroimaging data for single subject prediction of diagnosis across various neuropsychiatric disorders, including schizophrenia.[50] However, limitations across these studies include limited sample sizes, feature selection bias, lack of external validation, incomplete reporting of results, and unfair comparison across studies. Furthermore, very few single observations have emerged that have sufficient effect sizes to effectively discriminate between psychiatric disorders, although imaging findings show robust, but nonspecific, differences between patients with psychotic disorders and healthy subjects.[51] Single imaging features are limited by their inability to capture the heterogeneity and complexity of multifactorial brain disorders, such as schizophrenia, which are likely not related to discrete lesions, but are likely disorders of distributed brain circuits.[52] Precisely for this reason, machine learning approaches using multivariate imaging data for diagnosis in psychiatric disorders have shown promise. Modern data sharing models and data-intensive machine learning methodologies such as deep learning should be encouraged.[53]

The challenge in developing reliable diagnostic neuroimaging biomarkers for psychotic disorders may at least in part be related to current limitations in psychiatric nosology, with the disorders being distinguished based on symptom clusters rather than based on their underlying neurobiology. In a way, testing the diagnostic value of neuroimaging in psychiatric disorders is akin to comparing chest radiographs across groups defined by symptoms such as cough and breathlessness, rather than laboratory data (such as sputum microscopy). Testing the diagnostic value of imaging data may be more valuable across biologically defined subtypes than across symptom-based categories of psychotic disorders.[54,55] Notably, the work by Sun and colleagues[55] has been groundbreaking; it is the first study to parse the psychiatric disorders based on MR imaging in conjunction with and unsupervised machine learning technique and algorithm.

OUTCOME PREDICTION IN CLINICALLY HIGH-RISK INDIVIDUALS

Most individuals who develop psychosis (ie, 80%–90%) first experience a prodromal phase characterized by subthreshold symptoms, cognitive difficulties, and functional decline.[56] Identifying individuals at risk for psychosis at this early stage opens up opportunities for early intervention, which may ameliorate outcomes in youth prone to psychosis. The prodromal or high-risk stage is known with slight variations in clinical features as the clinical high risk, ultra-high risk, or at-risk mental state. The syndrome is diagnosed using clinical interviews that have been shown to have a prognostic accuracy comparable with other tests in preventive medicine.[57] However, their accuracy is mediated mainly by their ability to rule out psychosis, rather than their ability to differentiate among high-risk individuals in terms of outcomes. Given these drawbacks and the limitations of current treatments for psychosis, there is a need for improved outcome prediction in high-risk youth.

Neuroimaging data, on their own or in addition to clinical data, may contribute to improved prediction of psychosis in high-risk individuals.[58] There are 2 broad types of studies examining imaging biomarkers for psychosis in at-risk cohorts. The first type are cross-sectional studies of baseline imaging data in high-risk individuals who subsequently develop psychosis (ie, converters) as compared with those who do not (nonconverters). These studies suggest that converters show a number of structural and functional brain abnormalities as compared with nonconverters and controls, including gray matter changes in frontal, temporal, and cingulate cortices[59,60]; decreased integrity of striatal and (medial) temporal white matter[61]; aberrant language-related activation in frontal, temporal, and striatal regions[62]; and changes in functional connectivity and network organization.[63,64] The second type are machine learning studies that use a prediction model to separate converters from nonconverters and combine this with some type of cross-validation to estimate how the results of the model would generalize to an independent sample. For example, leave-one-out cross-validation leaves out 1 subject per run and classifies that individual subject using a model created from all other participants. Because this type of analysis facilitates outcome prediction based on individual patient data, it may in the future become useful in a clinical setting. Machine learning studies have shown considerable accuracy (ie, exceeding 80%) in separating converters from nonconverters, with classifiers relying mostly on gray and white matter changes in cingulate, frontal, and temporal cortex[65,66]; subcortical volumes of thalamus, amygdala, striatum, and cerebellum[67]; and

surface area changes involving mainly frontal, temporal, and parietal cortices.[67,68]

There is clearly a need for improved prediction of psychosis in clinical as well as familial high-risk youth, which may be achieved through the application of neuroimaging and machine-learning methods. Recent studies using these methods in high-risk cohorts suggest that neuroimaging predictors of psychosis include measures of brain structure, functional activation, and connectivity of predominantly the frontal, temporal, and cingulate cortex.

PREDICTION OF TREATMENT RESPONSE AND OUTCOME IN SCHIZOPHRENIA

Imaging technology can highlight observable differences in brain structure and function associated with treatment response. Hence, various factors at the molecular, functional and structural level may provide clues to predict treatment response in schizophrenia. Predictors of response to antipsychotic medication have been mostly studied using PET and MR imaging.

Pharmacologic treatments of first-episode psychosis or schizophrenia mainly target the dopamine synthesis pathway in the brain. At the molecular level, evidence suggests that individuals experiencing a first episode of psychosis or with a diagnosis of schizophrenia exhibit elevated striatal dopamine synthesis, and that individuals with greater striatal dopamine synthesis are more responsive to antipsychotic treatments.[69,70] At the functional level, greater response to antipsychotic medication in schizophrenia has also been associated with greater brain activation at baseline in the anterior cingulate cortex, temporal–parietal junction, and superior temporal gyrus.[71] Patients who respond to antipsychotic treatment also exhibit increased baseline amplitude of low-frequency fluctuations in the left postcentral gyrus/inferior parietal lobule relative to nonresponders.[72]

In addition to the suggested functional biomarkers of treatment response, spatial distribution information from brain tissue data acquired using structural MR imaging scans can also distinguish first episode psychosis patients who respond to treatment from those who do not.[73] Furthermore, there is evidence that a decreased gray matter volume as well as an abnormal reduction in gyrification (hypogyria) across multiple brain regions are associated with poor antipsychotic treatment response.[74,75] In contrast, studies investigating whether white matter connectivity in patients with schizophrenia is predictive of antipsychotic treatment response have shown inconsistent results. For instance, studies have reported higher FA in frontal regions to be associated with greater response to antipsychotic treatment, but some report a positive association,[76] although others report a negative association.[77]

In the search for potential predictors for non-pharmacologic treatment response in individuals with schizophrenia, structural brain markers have been identified as potential predictors of treatment response regarding cognitive remediation therapy and cognitive–behavioral therapy. Keshavan and colleagues[78] investigated the impact of cortical reserve as a structural brain predictor of cognitive improvement after cognitive remediation therapy. Baseline cortical surface area and gray matter volume predicted greater improvements in social cognition 1 year after cognitive remediation therapy. Similarly, Guimond and colleagues[79] observed a positive association between greater cortical reserve in the left prefrontal cortex at baseline and improved use of memory strategies after cognitive remediation therapy. Interestingly, greater gray matter volume in the prefrontal cortex, observed before therapy, is also associated with a considerable amelioration of positive symptoms following cognitive–behavioral therapy in individuals with schizophrenia.[80] Cortical reserve thus seems to predict cognitive and clinical outcomes after cognitive remediation therapy and behavioral therapy. This cortical reserve could reflect the level of neuroplasticity available in individuals with schizophrenia, thereby predisposing them to benefit from these types of therapies. If these findings are replicated, the results could provide further justification for combining cognitive remediation therapy or cognitive behavioral therapy with other approaches (ie, physical activity or brain stimulation) that could enhance brain plasticity.

Studies show that greater striatal dopamine synthesis, enlarged gray matter volume, and normal gyrification as well as increased brain activity in frontoparietal regions are potential markers of an individual's positive response to pharmacologic treatment in schizophrenia. There is less consistent evidence on brain markers associated with nonpharmacologic treatment response in schizophrenia, but greater gray matter volume and thickness in the prefrontal cortex could be predictive of a better response to nonpharmacologic treatment. Nonetheless, more research in this area is essential. A better understanding of neuroimaging biomarkers of treatment response could assist the development of more personalized treatments for people with schizophrenia. Hence, such biomarkers of treatment response may eventually guide targeted clinical decisions based on neuroimaging data.

CHALLENGES AND WAYS FORWARD

Neuroimaging literature accumulated over the last 4 decades has shed considerable light on the pathophysiology of schizophrenia. As it may be seen in **Table 1**, several observations are emerging from a variety of imaging techniques that provide a composite picture of the pathophysiological substrate of the heterogeneous syndrome we call schizophrenia. However, many large gaps in knowledge exist. There are numerous reasons for this, including the study of variable populations, methodological limitations, and small sample sizes. The limitations of our current neuroimaging approaches should also be considered as they still offer only a hazy view of the complex pathophysiology of this illness. Several novel imaging techniques are becoming available. One example is the use of synaptic vesicles glycoprotein as a ligand for PET imaging in a variety of psychiatric disorders.[81] Given the proposed synaptic abnormalities in schizophrenia this might become a powerful tool to investigate the pathophysiology of schizophrenia in the near future. In addition, neuromelanin MR imaging is now being used to examine dopamine release and has been found to show excessive dopamine in the substantia nigra of patients with schizophrenia.[82] While, Cassidy and colleagues[83] did not observe significant group differences between patients with schizophrenia and controls, they observed correlation with neuromelanin concentration, dopamine levels, and severity of psychosis in schizophrenia.[83] Another novel technique is neurite orientation dispersion and density imaging, which has shown altered gray matter microstructure in schizophrenia.[84]

A new area of investigation involving the integration of imaging data with genetic variations has been informative in revealing the association of genetic variations with structural, chemical, and functional brain changes observed in a given illness. Because these investigations are data driven and hypothesis free, large samples with adequate power are desirable along with corrections for multiple hypothesis testing.[85] Large-scale imaging data can be used to generate target phenotypes for discovery-based genetic associations, for example, databases such as the Enhancing Neuroimaging Genetics through Meta-Analysis showed common variants associated with hippocampal structural abnormalities.[86] Such efforts provide hints into the

Table 1
Summary of the proposed pathophysiological domains, imaging modalities, main findings and emerging approaches in the schizophrenia literature

	Hypothesized Measures	Imaging Modality	Frequently Replicated Findings in Schizophrenia	Emerging Approaches
Brain structure	Gray matter White matter tracts Synapse and neurite integrity	Structural MR imaging DTI	Widespread gray and white matter deficits, in particular in prefrontal and temporal regions, larger ventricles	Machine learning analyses NODDI, synaptic vesicle imaging High field MR imaging (7T) Shape analyses
Brain function	Cerebral blood flow Resting-state brain function Task-related brain function Neuroinflammation	PET, SPECT, Resting state fMR imaging, ASL, Task fMR imaging	Prefrontal hypoperfusion Altered function of default mode networks Altered task-related activation of prefrontal and temporal regions	Pseudocontinuous ASL Free water DTI
Brain connectivity	Long and short range connectivity, connectome organization	fMR imaging, DTI	Decreased long and short range connectivity Reduced connectome efficiency and altered modularity	Graph theory approaches
Brain chemistry	Dopamine Serotonin Glutamate GABA Neuropil integrity Neuropil synthesis and metabolism	PET PET, MRS ^{1}H MRS ^{1}H MRS, PET ^{1}H MRS ^{31}P MRS	Increased presynaptic dopamine Variable alterations in regional glutamate and GABA levels Reductions in N-acetyl aspartate Alterations in membrane phospholipid metabolites	High field MRS (7T) Neuromelanin MR imaging to investigate dopamine
Genetics	Multifactorial, polygenic	Structural MR imaging, DTI	Common variants associated with human hippocampal and intracranial volumes	Imaging genomics

Abbreviations: ASL, arterial spin labeling; DTI, diffusion tensor imaging; GABA, gamma aminobutyric acid; NODDI, neurite orientation dispersion and density imaging; PET, positron emission tomography.

pathophysiologic mechanisms and quantitative trait loci while controlling for false positives. This approach is being extended to study other genetic mechanisms such as epigenetics, gene–gene interactions, and gene–environment interactions.[87]

Although all these approaches will clearly shed considerable light on our understanding of schizophrenia, progress will also depend on a better elucidation of our current diagnostic system, which is still symptom based.[54] It is also critical that researchers pay careful attention to issues of reproducibility, effect sizes, specificity and sensitivity. Multisite consortia for large scale data collection, open data sharing approach, as well as rigorous methodology are likely to contribute to progress in the field.

At this time, the clinical value of imaging tools for diagnosis is limited apart from identifying organic brain pathologies in a small proportion of individuals with secondary psychoses. Nonetheless, there may be some value for imaging techniques to provide prediction of outcome. Imaging approaches may allow enhanced prediction or monitoring of therapeutic outcomes of treatments, such as pharmacologic agents, cognitive remediation, and neuromodulation. Similar to neurologic disorders, psychiatric disorders are more likely to be related to distributed neural network dysfunctions than discrete lesions.[88] For this reason, multivariate analysis of multimodal imaging datasets using machine learning approaches may offer better diagnostic and predictive value in schizophrenia and other psychiatric disorders at the individual level. Notably with the technical advancement, psychoradiology is showing promise from this perspective.[12,13,89]

ACKNOWLEDGMENTS

This work was supported by NIMH grants MH 78113 (M.S. Keshavan), MH112584 and MH115026 (K.M. Prasad), the Emerging Research Innovators in Mental Health Award from the IMHR (S. Guimond), a KL2/Catalyst Medical Research Investigator from Harvard Catalyst (P. Lizano), and the European Union's Horizon 2020 research and innovation program under Marie Sklodowska-Curie grant agreement No 749201 (G. Collin).

REFERENCES

1. Lieberman JA, First MB. Psychotic disorders. N Engl J Med 2018;379(3):270–80.
2. American Psychiatric Association. Diagnostic and statistical manual of mental disorders (5th edition.). Arlington (VA): American Psychiatric Association; 2013.
3. Seidman LJ, Mirsky AF. Evolving notions of schizophrenia as a developmental neurocognitive disorder. J Int Neuropsychol Soc 2017;23(9–10): 881–92.
4. Weinberger DR. Implications of normal brain development for the pathogenesis of schizophrenia. Arch Gen Psychiatry 1987;44(7):660–9.
5. Kelly S, Jahanshad N, Zalesky A, et al. Widespread white matter microstructural differences in schizophrenia across 4322 individuals: results from the ENIGMA Schizophrenia DTI Working Group. Mol Psychiatry 2018;23(5):1261–9.
6. Collin G, Keshavan MS. Connectome development and a novel extension to the neurodevelopmental model of schizophrenia. Dialogues Clin Neurosci 2018;20(2):101–11.
7. Glantz LA, Lewis DA. Decreased dendritic spine density on prefrontal cortical pyramidal neurons in schizophrenia. Arch Gen Psychiatry 2000;57(1): 65–73.
8. Lieberman JA. Is schizophrenia a neurodegenerative disorder? A clinical and neurobiological perspective. Biol Psychiatry 1999;46(6):729–39.
9. van Erp TGM, Hibar DP, Rasmussen JM, et al. Subcortical brain volume abnormalities in 2028 individuals with schizophrenia and 2540 healthy controls via the ENIGMA consortium. Mol Psychiatry 2016;21(4):585.
10. van Erp TGM, Walton E, Hibar DP, et al. Cortical brain abnormalities in 4474 individuals with schizophrenia and 5098 control subjects via the enhancing neuro imaging genetics through meta analysis (ENIGMA) consortium. Biol Psychiatry 2018;84(9): 644–54.
11. Friston KJ. Dysfunctional connectivity in schizophrenia. World Psychiatry 2002;1(2):66–71.
12. Huang X, Gong Q, Sweeney JA, et al. Progress in psychoradiology, the clinical application of psychiatric neuroimaging. Br J Radiol 2019;92(1101): 20181000.
13. Lui S, Zhou XJ, Sweeney JA, et al. Psychoradiology: the frontier of neuroimaging in psychiatry. Radiology 2016;281(2):357–72.
14. Gong Q. Response to Sarpal et al.: importance of neuroimaging biomarkers for treatment development and clinical practice. Am J Psychiatry 2016; 173(7):733–4.
15. Danhong W, Meiling L, Meiyun W, et al. Individual-specific functional connectivity markers track dimensional and categorical features of psychotic illness. Mol Psychiatry 2018. https://doi.org/10. 1038/s41380-018-0276-1.
16. Kubicki M, Shenton ME. Diffusion Tensor Imaging findings and their implications in schizophrenia. Curr Opin Psychiatry 2014;27(3):179–84.
17. Zalesky A, Fornito A, Seal ML, et al. Disrupted axonal fiber connectivity in schizophrenia. Biol Psychiatry 2011;69(1):80–9.
18. Gong Q, Lui S, Sweeney JA. A selective review of cerebral abnormalities in patients with first-episode schizophrenia before and after treatment. Am J Psychiatry 2016;173(3):232–43.
19. Lui S, Deng W, Huang X, et al. Association of cerebral deficits with clinical symptoms in antipsychotic-naive first-episode schizophrenia: an optimized voxel-based morphometry and resting state functional connectivity study. Am J Psychiatry 2009;166(2):196–205.
20. Tregellas J. Connecting brain structure and function in schizophrenia. Am J Psychiatry 2009; 166(2):134–6.
21. Wheeler AL, Voineskos AN. A review of structural neuroimaging in schizophrenia: from connectivity

to connectomics. Front Hum Neurosci 2014;8(402): 653.

22. Pasternak O, Kelly S, Sydnor VJ, et al. Advances in microstructural diffusion neuroimaging for psychiatric disorders. Neuroimage 2018;182:259–82.

23. Ingvar DH, Franzén G. Abnormalities of cerebral blood flow distribution in patients with chronic schizophrenia. Acta Psychiatr Scand 1974;50(4): 425–62.

24. O'Connell RA, Van Heertum RL, Billick SB, et al. Single photon emission computed tomography (SPECT) with [123I]IMP in the differential diagnosis of psychiatric disorders. J Neuropsychiatry Clin Neurosci 1989;1(2):145–53.

25. Kishimoto H, Kuwahara H, Ohno S, et al. Three subtypes of chronic schizophrenia identified using 11C-glucose positron emission tomography. Psychiatry Res 1987;21(4):285–92.

26. Sheppard G, Gruzelier J, Manchanda R, et al. 15O positron emission tomographic scanning in predominantly never-treated acute schizophrenic patients. Lancet 1983;2(8365–66):1448–52.

27. Logothetis NK. The underpinnings of the BOLD functional magnetic resonance imaging signal. J Neurosci 2003;23(10):3963–71.

28. Alsop DC, Detre JA, Golay X, et al. Recommended implementation of arterial spin-labeled perfusion MRI for clinical applications: a consensus of the ISMRM perfusion study group and the European consortium for ASL in dementia. Magn Reson Med 2015;73(1):102–16.

29. Hill K, Mann L, Laws KR, et al. Hypofrontality in schizophrenia: a meta-analysis of functional imaging studies. Acta Psychiatr Scand 2004;110(4):243–56.

30. Glahn DC, Ragland JD, Abramoff A, et al. Beyond hypofrontality: a quantitative meta-analysis of functional neuroimaging studies of working memory in schizophrenia. Hum Brain Mapp 2005;25(1):60–9.

31. Kühn S, Gallinat J. Resting-state brain activity in schizophrenia and major depression: a quantitative meta-analysis. Schizophr Bull 2013;39(2):358–65.

32. Guimarães TM, Machado-de-Sousa JP, Crippa JAS, et al. Arterial spin labeling in patients with schizophrenia: a systematic review. Archives of Clinical Psychiatry (São Paulo) 2016;43(6):151–6.

33. Stone JM, Davis JM, Leucht S, et al. Cortical dopamine D2/D3 receptors are a common site of action for antipsychotic drugs–an original patient data meta-analysis of the SPECT and PET in vivo receptor imaging literature. Schizophr Bull 2009;35(4): 789–97.

34. Abi-Dargham A, Rodenhiser J, Printz D, et al. Increased baseline occupancy of D2 receptors by dopamine in schizophrenia. Proc Natl Acad Sci U S A 2000;97(14):8104–9.

35. Laruelle M, Abi-Dargham A, Gil R, et al. Increased dopamine transmission in schizophrenia:

relationship to illness phases. Biol Psychiatry 1999; 46(1):56–72.

36. Zakzanis KK, Hansen KT. Dopamine D2 densities and the schizophrenic brain. Schizophr Res 1998; 32(3):201–6.

37. Chen KC, Yang YK, Howes O, et al. Striatal dopamine transporter availability in drug-naive patients with schizophrenia: a case-control SPECT study with [(99m)Tc]-TRODAT-1 and a meta-analysis. Schizophr Bull 2013;39(2):378–86.

38. Fusar-Poli P, Meyer-Lindenberg A. Striatal presynaptic dopamine in schizophrenia, part I: meta-analysis of dopamine active transporter (DAT) density. Schizophr Bull 2013;39(1):22–32.

39. Nikolaus S, Müller H-W, Hautzel H. Different patterns of 5-HT receptor and transporter dysfunction in neuropsychiatric disorders–a comparative analysis of in vivo imaging findings. Rev Neurosci 2016; 27(1):27–59.

40. Poels EMP, Kegeles LS, Kantrowitz JT, et al. Imaging glutamate in schizophrenia: review of findings and implications for drug discovery. Mol Psychiatry 2014;19(1):20–9.

41. Schür RR, Draisma LWR, Wijnen JP, et al. Brain GABA levels across psychiatric disorders: a systematic literature review and meta-analysis of (1) H-MRS studies. Hum Brain Mapp 2016;37(9):3337–52.

42. Egerton A, Modinos G, Ferrera D, et al. Neuroimaging studies of GABA in schizophrenia: a systematic review with meta-analysis. Transl Psychiatry 2017; 7(6):e1147.

43. Frankle WG, Cho RY, Prasad KM, et al. In vivo measurement of GABA transmission in healthy subjects and schizophrenia patients. Am J Psychiatry 2015; 172(11):1148–59.

44. Marsman A, van den Heuvel MP, Klomp DWJ, et al. Glutamate in schizophrenia: a focused review and meta-analysis of ^{1}H-MRS studies. Schizophr Bull 2013;39(1):120–9.

45. Merritt K, Egerton A, Kempton MJ, et al. Nature of glutamate alterations in schizophrenia: a meta-analysis of proton magnetic resonance spectroscopy studies. JAMA Psychiatry 2016;73(7): 665–74.

46. Reddy R, Keshavan MS. Phosphorus magnetic resonance spectroscopy: its utility in examining the membrane hypothesis of schizophrenia. Prostaglandins Leukot Essent Fatty Acids 2003;69(6):401–5.

47. Du F, Cooper AJ, Thida T, et al. In vivo evidence for cerebral bioenergetic abnormalities in schizophrenia measured using 31P magnetization transfer spectroscopy. JAMA Psychiatry 2014;71(1):19–27.

48. Lubman DI, Velakoulis D, McGorry PD, et al. Incidental radiological findings on brain magnetic resonance imaging in first-episode psychosis and chronic schizophrenia. Acta Psychiatr Scand 2002; 106(5):331–6.

49. Freudenreich O, Schulz SC, Goff DC. Initial medical work-up of first-episode psychosis: a conceptual review. Early Interv Psychiatry 2009;3(1):10–8.

50. Rozycki M, Satterthwaite TD, Koutsouleris N, et al. Multisite machine learning analysis provides a robust structural imaging signature of schizophrenia detectable across diverse patient populations and within individuals. Schizophr Bull 2018;44(5):1035–44.

51. Fusar-Poli P, Meyer-Lindenberg A. Forty years of structural imaging in psychosis: promises and truth. Acta Psychiatr Scand 2016;134(3):207–24.

52. Atluri G, Padmanabhan K, Fang G, et al. Complex biomarker discovery in neuroimaging data: finding a needle in a haystack. Neuroimage Clin 2013;3:123–31.

53. Arbabshirani MR, Plis S, Sui J, et al. Single subject prediction of brain disorders in neuroimaging: promises and pitfalls. Neuroimage 2017;145(Pt B):137–65.

54. Clementz BA, Sweeney JA, Hamm JP, et al. Identification of distinct psychosis biotypes using brain-based biomarkers. Am J Psychiatry 2016;173(4):373–84.

55. Sun H, Lui S, Yao L, et al. Two patterns of white matter abnormalities in medication-naive patients with first-episode schizophrenia revealed by diffusion tensor imaging and cluster analysis. JAMA Psychiatry 2015;72:678–86.

56. Cannon TD, Chung Y, He G, et al. Progressive reduction in cortical thickness as psychosis develops: a multisite longitudinal neuroimaging study of youth at elevated clinical risk. Biol Psychiatry 2015;77(2):147–57.

57. Fusar-Poli P, Cappucciati M, Rutigliano G, et al. At risk or not at risk? A meta-analysis of the prognostic accuracy of psychometric interviews for psychosis prediction. World Psychiatry 2015;14(3):322–32.

58. McGuire P, Dazzan P. Does neuroimaging have a role in predicting outcomes in psychosis? World Psychiatry 2017;16(2):209–10.

59. Koutsouleris N, Meisenzahl EM, Davatzikos C, et al. Use of neuroanatomical pattern classification to identify subjects in at-risk mental states of psychosis and predict disease transition. Arch Gen Psychiatry 2009;66(7):700–12.

60. Mechelli A, Riecher-Rössler A, Meisenzahl EM, et al. Neuroanatomical abnormalities that predate the onset of psychosis: a multicenter study. Arch Gen Psychiatry 2011;68(5):489–95.

61. Bloemen OJN, de Koning MB, Schmitz N, et al. White-matter markers for psychosis in a prospective ultra-high-risk cohort. Psychol Med 2010;40(8):1297–304.

62. Sabb FW, van Erp TGM, Hardt ME, et al. Language network dysfunction as a predictor of outcome in youth at clinical high risk for psychosis. Schizophr Res 2010;116(2–3):173–83.

63. Cao H, Chén OY, Chung Y, et al. Cerebello-thalamo-cortical hyperconnectivity as a state-independent functional neural signature for psychosis prediction and characterization. Nat Commun 2018;9(1):3836–9.

64. Collin G, Seidman LJ, Keshavan MS, et al. Functional connectome organization predicts conversion to psychosis in clinical high-risk youth from the SHARP program. Mol Psychiatry 2018;41:801–10.

65. Koutsouleris N, Riecher-Rössler A, Meisenzahl EM, et al. Detecting the psychosis prodrome across high-risk populations using neuroanatomical biomarkers. Schizophr Bull 2015;41(2):471–82.

66. Koutsouleris N, Schmitt GJE, Gaser C, et al. Neuroanatomical correlates of different vulnerability states for psychosis and their clinical outcomes. Br J Psychiatry 2009;195(3):218–26.

67. de Wit S, Ziermans TB, Nieuwenhuis M, et al. Individual prediction of long-term outcome in adolescents at ultra-high risk for psychosis: applying machine learning techniques to brain imaging data. Hum Brain Mapp 2017;38(2):704–14.

68. Kambeitz-Ilankovic L, Meisenzahl EM, Cabral C, et al. Prediction of outcome in the psychosis prodrome using neuroanatomical pattern classification. Schizophr Res 2016;173(3):159–65.

69. Demjaha A, Murray RM, McGuire PK, et al. Dopamine synthesis capacity in patients with treatment-resistant schizophrenia. Am J Psychiatry 2012;169(11):1203–10.

70. Jauhar S, Veronese M, Nour MM, et al. Determinants of treatment response in first-episode psychosis: an 18F-DOPA PET study. Mol Psychiatry 2018. https://doi.org/10.1038/s41380-018-0042-4.

71. Shafritz KM, Ikuta T, Greene A, et al. Frontal lobe functioning during a simple response conflict task in first-episode psychosis and its relationship to treatment response. Brain Imaging Behav 2019;13(2):541–53.

72. Cui L-B, Cai M, Wang X-R, et al. Prediction of early response to overall treatment for schizophrenia: a functional magnetic resonance imaging study. Brain Behav 2019;9(2):e01211.

73. Mourao-Miranda J, Reinders AATS, Rocha-Rego V, et al. Individualized prediction of illness course at the first psychotic episode: a support vector machine MRI study. Psychol Med 2012;42(5):1037–47.

74. Arango C, Breier A, McMahon R, et al. The relationship of clozapine and haloperidol treatment response to prefrontal, hippocampal, and caudate brain volumes. Am J Psychiatry 2003;160(8):1421–7.

75. Molina V, Reig S, Sarramea F, et al. Anatomical and functional brain variables associated with clozapine

response in treatment-resistant schizophrenia. Psychiatry Res 2003;124(3):153–61.

76. Reis Marques T, Taylor H, Chaddock C, et al. White matter integrity as a predictor of response to treatment in first episode psychosis. Brain 2014;137(Pt 1):172–82.

77. Kim M-K, Kim B, Lee KS, et al. White-matter connectivity related to paliperidone treatment response in patients with schizophrenia. J Psychopharmacol 2016;30(3):294–302.

78. Keshavan MS, Nasrallah HA, Tandon R. Schizophrenia, "Just the Facts" 6. Moving ahead with the schizophrenia concept: from the elephant to the mouse. Schizophr Res 2011;127(1–3):3–13.

79. Guimond S, Béland S, Lepage M. Strategy for Semantic Association Memory (SESAME) training: effects on brain functioning in schizophrenia. Psychiatry Res Neuroimaging 2018;271:50–8.

80. Premkumar P, Fannon D, Sapara A, et al. Orbitofrontal cortex, emotional decision-making and response to cognitive behavioural therapy for psychosis. Psychiatry Res 2015;231(3):298–307.

81. Cai Z, Li S, Matuskey D, et al. PET imaging of synaptic density: a new tool for investigation of neuropsychiatric diseases. Neurosci Lett 2019;691:44–50.

82. Watanabe Y, Tanaka H, Tsukabe A, et al. Neuromelanin magnetic resonance imaging reveals increased dopaminergic neuron activity in the substantia nigra of patients with schizophrenia. PLoS One 2014;9(8):e104619.

83. Cassidy CM, Zucca FA, Girgis RR, et al. Neuromelanin-sensitive MRI as a noninvasive proxy measure of dopamine function in the human brain. Proc Natl Acad Sci U S A 2019;116(11):5108–17.

84. Nazeri A, Mulsant BH, Rajji TK, et al. Gray matter neuritic microstructure deficits in schizophrenia and bipolar disorder. Biol Psychiatry 2017;82(10):726–36.

85. Carter CS, Bearden CE, Bullmore ET, et al. Enhancing the informativeness and replicability of imaging genomics studies. Biol Psychiatry 2017;82(3):157–64.

86. Stein JL, Medland SE, Vasquez AA, et al. Identification of common variants associated with human hippocampal and intracranial volumes. Nat Genet 2012;44(5):552–61.

87. Mufford MS, Stein DJ, Dalvie S, et al. Neuroimaging genomics in psychiatry-a translational approach. Genome Med 2017;9(1):102–12.

88. Perez DL, Keshavan MS, Scharf JM, et al. Bridging the great divide: what can neurology learn from psychiatry? J Neuropsychiatry Clin Neurosci 2018;30(4):271–8.

89. Lei D, Pinaya WHL, van Amelsvoort T, et al. Detecting schizophrenia at the level of the individual: relative diagnostic value of whole-brain images, connectome-wide functional connectivity and graph-based metrics. Psychol Med 2019;1–10. https://doi.org/10.1017/S0033291719001934.

Widespread Morphometric Abnormalities in Major Depression
Neuroplasticity and Potential for Biomarker Development

Cynthia H.Y. Fu, MD, PhD[a,b,*], Yong Fan, PhD[c], Christos Davatzikos, PhD[c]

KEYWORDS

- MR imaging • Psychoradiology • Machine learning • Neuroplasticity • Anterior cingulate
- Hippocampus • Antidepressant • Psychotherapy

KEY POINTS

- Widespread morphometric abnormalities in depression reflect cytoarchitecture alterations in corticolimbic regions, including anterior cingulate, orbitofrontal, and middle frontal regions to lateral temporal and inferior parietal cortices, hippocampus, and cerebellum.
- Neural circuitries involved in emotion regulation, such as reward processing, attention and memory, overlap with the neural circuitries that control the homeostatic stress response systems, which are disrupted in major depression.
- MR imaging observable changes in hippocampal structure, and in other cortical and subcortical regions, reflect the complex inter-relationships of neurotoxic and neuroplastic cellular effects.
- Multivariate pattern analysis offers the potential to develop biomarkers to identify the biological subtypes that comprise major depression and predict clinical outcome.
- We would not expect perfect concordance in classification results with current diagnostic criteria because they do not reflect specific biological pathophysiologies.

INTRODUCTION

Major depression is a common mental health disorder, affecting about 350 million persons worldwide with a lifetime prevalence of around 15% of the population,[1] and is predicted to be the leading contributor to the global burden of disease.[2] The disorder is characterized by a prolonged low mood or an inability to experience usual feelings of enjoyment along with changes in neurovegetative symptoms, such as fatigue and disturbances in appetite, sleep, and psychomotor functioning, as well as cognitive impairments, feelings of guilt, and, for some, suicidal ideation with intent. The disorder is characterized by impairments in mood, behavior, and cognition, which are associated with neurobiological abnormalities. However, the diagnosis is

Disclosure Statement: None.
[a] School of Psychology, University of East London, Arthur Edwards Building, Water Lane, London E15 4LZ, UK;
[b] Centre for Affective Disorders, Institute of Psychiatry, Psychology and Neuroscience, King's College London, London, UK; [c] Center for Biomedical Image Computing and Analytics, Department of Radiology, Perelman School of Medicine, University of Pennsylvania, Philadelphia, PA 19104, USA
* Corresponding author. School of Psychology, University of East London, Arthur Edwards Building, Water Lane, London E15 4LZ, UK.
E-mail address: c.fu@uel.ac.uk

currently based solely on clinical features.[3,4] This is problematic because the diagnosis is made only from self-report symptoms and observable behaviors. Many phenotypic combinations are possible, which are not linked to a specific pathophysiology. Based on current classification systems, major depression is a heterogeneous syndrome that is not linked to etiology.

Furthermore, treatment selection is based on trial and error. The most common first-line treatments are antidepressant medications and psychological therapies. It typically takes weeks before clinical improvement is evident, and yet the remission rate is only about 30% after a full 3-month treatment trial.[5] The course of the disorder typically consists of recurrent episodes, although it may be chronic with persistent symptoms for some patients despite a series of treatment trials.[6] There is significant heterogeneity in the clinical outcomes and longitudinal course of the disorder, but it is not possible to predict the likelihood of response for a given treatment at the level of the individual. Currently, there are no biological markers that can help to identify depression or to predict clinical outcome.

Notwithstanding limitations in diagnosis and treatment selection, neural alterations have been observed consistently in neuroimaging studies. Neuroimaging markers offer a promising biological measure, which can aid in identifying depression and predict clinical outcome because no other measure to date has demonstrated the same level of accuracy at the level of the individual. Heritability estimates for major depression are low, around 37%, in contrast with bipolar disorder and schizophrenia, which have consistently high heritability estimates of up to 90%.[7] Although environmental risk factors are known to have a strong contribution, the mechanism of how genetic risk variants lead to the development of an acute depressive episode is unclear,[8] and no genetic predictors of clinical response been identified at the level of the individual.[9,10]

WIDESPREAD MORPHOMETRIC ABNORMALITIES REFLECT CYTOARCHITECTURE ALTERATIONS

The term limbic lobe is derived from Latin, *limbus* for border, to refer to the brain structures located at the inferior rim of the neocortex and superior to the brainstem. Papez[11] proposed a circuit as the basis for emotion processing, composed of the hippocampus (subiculum), fornix, mamillary bodies, anterior nucleus of the thalamus, cingulate gyrus, parahippocampal gyrus, and entorhinal cortex, which has since also become recognized

for its role in memory formation, in particular episodic memory.[12] MacLean[13] proposed the limbic system to be a functionally integrated set of regions that underlie emotion processing and motivation. Although the regions that comprise the limbic system continue to be debated, they generally include the orbitofrontal, cingulate and insular cortices, hippocampal formation, and amygdala, as well as thalamus, hypothalamus and basal ganglia.[14]

Genetic and environmental factors that lead to major depressive disorder (MDD) are expressed in neural structure and function. A range of sometimes contradictory findings have been reported, owing in part to heterogeneity in sample characteristics, such as medication status, the presence of comorbid disorders, and the form of depression, including treatment-resistant depression, in addition to heterogeneity in methodologies in data acquisition, processing, and analysis. Meta-analyses seek to quantitatively incorporate the collective findings to identify the strongest effects. Widespread volumetric reductions in gray matter have been demonstrated in meta-analyses in MDD. Affected regions include corticolimbic circuits involved in emotion regulation as well as more broadly in cortical and subcortical regions,[15–19] which can be observed in the first depressive episode[15,20,21] and reflect neuronal and glial reductions.[22–24]

Recent meta-analyses have sought to address potential biases and to combine datasets to take into account subtle effects that may not have achieve statistical significance in small samples. Atkinson and colleagues[16] performed a meta-analysis that included studies of recurrent MDD that was not treatment resistant and pooled both voxel-based morphometry and region of interest-based analyses together with reports of no significant differences in gray matter volume or density in MDD (n = 1341) and healthy (n = 1364) participants. Wise and colleagues[19] conducted a meta-analysis that combined between-group voxel-based morphometry data in MDD (n = 1736) and healthy (n = 2365) participants from individual studies, and Schmaal and colleagues[15,18] integrated measures of cortical thickness and surface area estimates from individual MDD (n = 1902 adults) and healthy (n = 7658) participants across sites. Gray matter volume is a product of the surface area and cortical thickness, which have distinct genetic and developmental origins.[25] Measures of regional gray matter, including gray matter density, complement measures of its components, although surface area has a substantially greater contribution than cortical thickness.[26]

Gray matter volumetric reductions have been observed in the prefrontal cortex encompassing the bilateral anterior cingulate cortices (Brodmann areas [BAs] 24 and 32), medial regions including superior medial frontal (BA 32) to medial orbitofrontal cortices (BA 11), superior frontal gyri, as well as lateral regions in the middle frontal (BA 46) and inferior frontal cortices (BA 47), which are involved in executive function and emotion regulation.[15,16,19] Cortical volumetric decreases extend into the bilateral insula, involved in interoceptive awareness, as well as in postcentral, temporal, and inferior parietal cortices, and the cerebellum. Subcortical regions include the thalamus, caudate, and putamen, although with mixed findings.[16,19] Most regions have demonstrated decrease in surface area as well as cortical thickness, whereas some regions, including the inferior parietal cortices and supramarginal gyri, primarily show decreases in cortical thickness.[15]

Structural and functional alterations in the anterior cingulate cortex and amygdala have been widely observed in MDD. Reduced anterior cingulate volumes have been observed in medication naïve MDD in the first episode and when medication free later in the illness course, which avoids potential effects of medication,[27,28] and decreased amygdala volumes have been reported, although with inconsistent findings.[29] The amygdala sends projections toward the subgenual anterior cingulate and in turn receives projections from dorsal cingulate cortex.[30] Voluntary emotional regulation is linked to suppression of amygdala activity though activation in pregenual and dorsal anterior cingulate as well as in middle frontal and orbitofrontal cortices.[31] Effective emotional regulation depends on the interplay between the anterior cingulate, prefrontal regions, and the amygdala, which is disrupted in MDD.[32]

One of the most consistent findings has been decreased hippocampal volumes bilaterally, with estimates in the range of 1% to 4%.[16–20] Hippocampal atrophy was initially identified in recurrent MDD, associated with total lifetime duration of depression[33,34] and multiple depressive episodes.[35] However, hippocampal atrophy has also observed in the first episode of depression,[20] in individuals with high familial risk of developing depression,[36] and in adolescents with early onset depression[37] in whom attenuated growth is linked to the onset of the first depressive episode.[38]

Decreased hippocampal volumes, however, are not specific to MDD because they are a feature in a many psychiatric disorders, including bipolar disorder, schizophrenia, obsessive–compulsive disorder, and borderline personality disorder.[39–44] Quantifying the distinct subfields that comprise hippocampal morphology can delineate the regional deformations that are characteristic as well as shared with other disorders. Deformations have been reported in the subiculum[45] and in the cornu ammonis (CA) subfields CA1 extending into CA2/3[45,46] as well as CA4,[46] and multiple depressive episodes are associated with a significant declines in subfield regional volumes.[42] Bipolar disorder may be associated with more prominent decreases in subfield volumes,[43] although with mixed findings,[40] whereas more extensive decreases seem to be present in schizophrenia and old age depression.[39,41,44,47]

In comparison with bipolar disorder, MDD is associated with common as well as distinct patterns of morphometric alterations.[19] Both disorders show decreased gray matter volume in the dorsomedial and ventromedial prefrontal cortices, which included the anterior cingulate, and bilateral insula, suggesting a common neuropathology to affective disorders. Greater decreases in the right middle frontal cortex, left hippocampus, along with parietal, temporal, and cerebellar regions were found in MDD relative to bipolar disorder, indicating a specificity to MDD that could aid in the development of biomarkers.[48]

ENDOGENOUS STRESS RESPONSE SYSTEMS, MONOAMINERGIC SYSTEMS, AND NEUROPLASTICITY

Neural circuitries involved in emotion regulation, such as reward processing, attention and memory, overlap with the neural circuitries that control the homeostatic stress response systems, which are disrupted in MDD. The hypothalamic–pituitary–adrenocortical (HPA) axis is an endogenous feedback circuit activated by perturbations in homeostasis. In addition to the HPA axis, there are many interacting endogenous stress response systems, including the autonomic nervous system, which generates immediate responses, for example, increased heart rate and blood pressure, through sympathetic and parasympathetic innervations, and the inflammatory cytokine systems. MDD is associated with elevated proinflammatory cytokine levels, in particular during an acute depressive episode as well as being a risk factor in itself in the development of MDD and a moderating factor in the association of childhood maltreatment with MDD.[49,50]

HPA axis hyperactivity is a well-replicated finding in MDD. HPA disturbances characterised by adrenal hypersecretion of glucocorticoids, namely, cortisol in humans, has been linked to hippocampal atrophy with evidence of neuronal loss, dendritic atrophy, and inhibition of neurogenesis in the hippocampus in animal models.[51] The hippocampus is a plastic brain structure with a pivotal role in memory and learning that is, responsive to adrenocortical, thyroid and gonadal hormones together with excitatory amino acid neurotransmitters through N-methyl-D-aspartate receptors.[51]

The MR imaging observable regional abnormalities reflect cytoarchitectonic alterations within a local neuroendocrine milieu that has systemic effects. Adrenocorticosteroid receptors in the prefrontal regions regulate glucocorticoid secretion in the HPA axis stress response circuit.[52] In animal studies, lesions in the dorsal division of the medial prefrontal cortex enhanced HPA glucocorticoid responses to psychogenic stressors, whereas lesions in the ventromedial division attenuated stress responses,[53] with comparable opposing effects on heart rate, in which the dorsal division decreased tachycardiac responses and the ventral division facilitated the effect.[54] The medial prefrontal cortex has distinct effects on the autonomic nervous system stress response systems as focal damage involving the anterior cingulate cortex in humans has been associated with impaired cardiovascular responses during cognitive effort despite preserved performance.[55]

Monoaminergic neurotransmitters, such as serotonin, dopamine, and noradrenaline, project into the medial prefrontal cortex with direct neural effects as well as modulator effects on psychogenic stress-induced HPA neuroendocrine responses. These effects are associated with distinct in vivo neurocognitive signals in MDD. Postmortem tissue studies indicate that alterations in innervation of medial prefrontal cortex could underlie reduced monoamine availability.[56–59] Changes in regional cerebral volumes after antidepressant treatment reflect cytoarchitectonic neuroplasticity effects, and early changes have been predictive of clinical outcome. Neuroplastic changes in serotonin (5-hydroxytryptamine) neurons in the ventromedial prefrontal cortex and dentate gyrus in the hippocampus have been associated with antidepressant effects in animal models.[60]

In humans, increased hippocampal volume observed after selective serotonin reuptake inhibitor (SSRI) antidepressant treatment could reflect cellular neuroplasticity.[61] Moreover, an early increase in hippocampal volume and in rostral anterior cingulate thickness after 1 week of treatment was predictive of improved clinical response to antidepressant treatment with serotonin and noradrenaline reuptake inhibitor antidepressant drugs, suggesting that neuroplastic cellular changes may occur early and are predictive of subsequent clinical efficacy.[62,63] Furthermore, decreased hippocampal gray matter in MDD in a current depressive episode, relative to healthy participants and MDD in remission, subsequently showed increased gray matter after SSRI antidepressant treatment,[61] perhaps representing a human in vivo correlate of cellular neurogenesis with SSRI pharmacologic treatment in animal models.[64]

MR imaging observable changes in hippocampal structure, as well as in other cortical and subcortical regions, reflect the complex interrelationships of neurotoxic and neuroplastic cellular effects. Persistent depressive symptoms have been associated with a progressive decrease in hippocampal volume,[65] and recurrent depressive episodes in MDD are associated with decreased hippocampal volumes and more extensive subregional deficits,[66] supporting neuroprogressive models of stress-related neural atrophy. Increases in hippocampal volume after antidepressant treatment in humans though reflect the potential for neuroplasticity.[61] Moreover, evidence of hippocampal atrophy preceding and present at disease onset also reflect complex neurodevelopmental mechanisms in the potential interactions of genetic vulnerability with environmental risk factors, such as childhood maltreatment and low socioeconomic status, during key periods in the trajectory of cortical and subcortical development leading to the onset of MDD.[20,67,68]

Advances in functional neuroimaging methods have provided enhanced resolution and capabilities to delineate the functional neural correlates in MDD. Initial studies examined performance-related effects associated with stimuli-induced responses to a specific task. A fundamental neuropsychological impairment in MDD is a mood-congruent processing bias toward negative valences in which ambiguous or positively valenced stimuli are perceived as negative, which is evident in a number of domain, including memory, attention, and perception.[69,70] Groenewold and colleagues[71] meta-analysis demonstrated that negative and positive stimuli are associated with opposing effects in limbic and visual processing regions, while there may be valence-specific effects in the prefrontal cortex. Negative stimuli were associated with increased activity in amygdala, anterior cingulate, parahippocampal and hippocampal regions, striatum and cerebellum, and reduced decreased in the left superior and middle frontal regions. Positive emotions were associated with opposing effects in the same regions along with increased activity in the orbitofrontal cortex. The findings consistent with models of emotion processing in MDD, which have proposed limbocortical dysregulation,[72] as well as a ventral system for production of emotion states, which includes the amygdala, insula, ventral anterior cingulate, orbitofrontal and ventrolateral prefrontal regions, and dorsal system underlying effortful regulation of emotion responses that includes the hippocampus, dorsal anterior cingulate, and middle frontal regions.[73] Meta-analysis further suggests that there are specific regions in the prefrontal cortex that distinguish positive and negative emotional valences.

Discerning the specific emotions that comprise a particular valence, for example, sadness, fear, disgust, or anger within the category of negative valence, offers the potential to determine whether there are distinct functional neurocircuitries in the clinical subtypes that comprise MDD and to distinguish MDD from comorbid disorders and the effects of concurrent symptoms, such as anxiety disorders and anxiety symptoms, which are common in MDD. A highly replicated finding in longitudinal pharmacologic treatment studies is that activity in the amygdala and ventral regions in the anterior cingulate cortex in response to sad facial expression is increased during an acute depressive episode and normalizes after antidepressant treatment.[74,75] This pattern in the amygdala response is specific to sad facial expressions.[76]

Similarly, in a prospective, longitudinal treatment study with cognitive–behavioral therapy, we found that increased amygdala activity to sad facial expressions in MDD during an acute depressive episode normalized after a course of treatment in comparison with healthy participants who underwent the same set of MR imaging scans.[77] Our meta-analysis of longitudinal treatment effects after psychotherapy found a significant group by time effect in the left rostral anterior cingulate in response to emotional stimuli, in which MDD participants showed increased activity following treatment while healthy participants showed a decrease in activity at the follow-up scan.[78] Ventral–rostral regions in the anterior cingulate have a regulatory function on emotion processing, as well as in reward processing and decision making, through interconnections with core emotion processing regions, in particular the amygdala.[79] MDD is associated with a bias toward negative affective valences, which is also evident in a decreased ability to disengage from negative stimuli.[80] Healthy emotion regulation is associated with suppression of amygdala activity through interconnections with the rostral and dorsal anterior cingulate and middle frontal cortices,

but the connectivity between the anterior cingulate and amygdala is impaired in MDD.[31,32] The observed increase in rostral anterior cingulate activity is suggestive of improvements in emotion regulation after a course of treatment with psychotherapy.

The number of longitudinal psychotherapy treatment studies in MDD, however, has been less than one-third of the number of longitudinal pharmacologic treatment studies.[81] Although combining MDD with other psychiatric disorders, including panic disorder, post-traumatic stress disorder, social anxiety disorder, and obsessive–compulsive disorder, and incorporating different forms of cognitive and emotion-based functional tasks, generates a larger sample size, a meta-analysis[82] of the combined disorders and combined cognitive and emotion-based tasks may confound the functional neural effects; for example, cognitive and emotional tasks are associated with differing and potentially opposing neural effects, such as on amygdala responsivity.[83]

NEUROIMAGING-BASED BIOMARKERS

Yet, MDD in its current form is a heterogeneous disorder that is not linked to etiology. Current diagnostic criteria are based solely on clinical features and many phenotypic combinations are possible. The widespread extent of structural volumetric reductions reflects the emotional, social, and cognitive impairments that are common in MDD. To identify an acute depressive episode in MDD and to predict clinical outcome are key clinical challenges.

Multivariate pattern analysis is able to integrate the spatially distributed, subtle alterations into models. From learning to categorize these models, it would be possible to then identify comparable models in novel brain imaging data. We demonstrated the ability to identify MDD at the level of the individual with proof-of-concept data using structural MR imaging and task-based functional MR imaging that included gray matter as well as white matter in the medial and superior frontal regions, superior parietal and inferior occipital gyri, and in the cerebellum, which was distinct from the pattern that was predictive of clinical outcome.[84–86] In the largest multisite sample to date, multiple classification subtype models were identified, which included a common pattern of altered connectivity that encompassed the ventromedial prefrontal, orbitofrontal and posterior cingulate cortices, insula, and subcortical regions, along with distinct patterns of functional connectivity and clinical symptom profiles in 4 subtypes with different profiles of clinical symptoms.[87]

Distinct patterns of classification have also been demonstrated in bipolar disorder and MDD in which decreased gray matter volumes in the anterior cingulate provided a greater contribution in MDD as supported by morphometric data.[19,88,89]

Increased anterior cingulate activity during an acute depressive episode before the initiation of treatment, has been consistently associated with a higher likelihood of a better clinical outcome. Our meta-analysis of neural predictors of clinical response found that the regional activity extended from the dorsal to rostral anterior cingulate into the medial prefrontal and orbitofrontal regions, whereas activity in the insula and striatum was predictive of a lower likelihood of clinical benefit from treatment.[81] Applying multivariate pattern analysis, the regional cerebral pattern that predicted clinical outcome before the initiation of treatment included greater gray matter density in the rostral anterior cingulate and posterior cingulate cortices, which increased the probability of a full clinical response and increased gray matter density in the orbitofrontal cortex increased the probability of persistent residual symptoms after pharmacologic treatment.[84–86]

The quality of the data and methodology in model development are essential inputs. Although the highest rates of classification have been achieved in treatment-resistant forms of MDD, the neural correlates are usually confounded by the potential effects of medication and a chronic course of illness. Developing models in MDD in an acute depressive episode that is medication-free could more accurately reflect the neural features that have not been confounded by effects of medication. We would not expect perfect concordance in the classification results with current diagnostic criteria, which do not reflect specific biological pathophysiologies. We expect that the development of biomarkers would be an iterative process in which the neuroimaging-based biomarkers are applied to specify potential pathophysiology.[48]

We propose that it is essential to address heterogeneity in the symptom profiles that make up the clinical disorder, the clinical outcomes for a given treatment (which reflects a combination of the inherent likelihood of response and the mechanisms of treatment), and the longitudinal course for individual patients. High dimensional clustering methods applied to dissect imaging heterogeneity are confounded by variations related to demographics and other factors that are not related to disease pathophysiology.[88] Recent literature has proposed 2 semisupervised learning methods in an attempt to address these confounds: CHIMERA[90] and HYDRA.[91] Both of these methods can be viewed as semisupervised clustering methods—they rely on well-defined groups of patients and controls; however, they let the data reveal patient subtypes based on the way in which they differ from healthy controls. Put simply, these methods do not cluster patients directly, which might be confounded by covariates such as age and sex, but they aim to cluster the differences between patients and healthy controls, which is more likely to yield disease subphenotypes.

CHIMERA is primarily generative, in which it assumes a statistical distribution of imaging features of the patient cohort that is, heterogeneous which is derived from the statistical distribution of healthy controls through a number of transformations that reflect the effects of underlying pathophysiologies that are also heterogeneous. Covariates are taken into account explicitly. CHIMERA is a probabilistic clustering approach that models pathologic processes through a combination of multiple regularized transformations from the healthy population to the MDD patient population. The populations are considered as point distributions that are matched by a variant of the coherent point drift algorithm, such that, for example, a 40-year-old woman with MDD would have been a 40-year-old healthy woman had she been spared the disorder. CHIMERA directly models these effects by seeking to identify the multiple imaging patterns that relate to disease effects to characterize disease heterogeneity.

HYDRA takes a similar approach, but from the discriminative angle. HYDRA applies a number of support vector machine hyperplanes to separate patients from health controls in which each hyperplane reflects one subtype. Covariates are first regressed out of the data, and the subtypes are captured by multiple linear hyperplanes, forming a convex polytope that separates 2 populations in which each face of the polytope defines a disease subtype. Both CHIMERA and HYDRA methods use cross-validation and split sample analyses to determine the optimal number of subtypes, and have been recently shown to elucidate heterogeneity in mild cognitive impairment and Alzheimer disease, and to associate neuroanatomical subtypes with clinical progression.[92] These methods have also revealed, for the first time, significant heterogeneity in neuroanatomical signatures of schizophrenia,[93] as well as in adolescents with internalizing symptoms.[94]

Data-driven, inductive modeling strategies would model the neuroanatomical patterns that make up MDD as a collection of directions of deviation from normal neuroanatomical patterns. Classification results in schizophrenia, mild cognitive impairment, and Alzheimer's disease demonstrate the potential of these methods to capture neuroanatomic heterogeneity from MR imaging data.[92,93] The approaches model the pathologic processes associated with MDD through a combination of multiple regularized transformations from the healthy control population to the patient population. The methods seek to identify multiple neuroanatomic patterns that relate to disease effects and to characterize disease heterogeneity. A deductive approach, such as reported clinical symptoms, would apply prior knowledge to identify the linear and nonlinear combinations of neuroanatomic features that correlate with clinical clusters, which could be a complementary process. A synergistic combination could bring together the data-driven inductive and symptom-based deductive approaches such that the clinical measures will be used in CHIMERA and HYDRA to inform the clustering.

SUMMARY

MDD is associated with widespread morphometric abnormalities extending from frontolimbic regions which reflect cytoarchitectural alterations believed to result from complex interrelationships of neurotoxic and neuroplastic cellular effects. Neural circuitries involved in emotion regulation overlap with the neural circuitries that control the homeostatic stress response systems, which are disrupted in MDD. Functional and structural effects have been observed after treatment with antidepressant medication as well as psychotherapy. Yet, current diagnostic criteria for MDD are based solely on clinical signs and symptoms, and many phenotypic combinations are possible. MDD in its current form is a heterogeneous disorder that is not linked to etiology. Identifying the neurobiological subtypes that comprise MDD and predicting clinical outcome are key clinical challenges. Applying multivariate pattern analysis offers the potential to identify the neurobiological subtypes that comprise MDD and predictors of clinical outcome at the level of the individual. It is essential to characterize disease heterogeneity in which a synergistic combination could incorporate data-driven inductive and symptom-based deductive approaches in an iterative process. In future, psychoradiology, a subdivision of neuroradiology, may also play an important role for enhancing our understanding of disease mechanisms and aiding clinical management in patients with depression.[95-98]

ACKNOWLEDGMENTS

Drs C. Davatzikos and Y. Fan acknowledge support from NIH grants AG054409 and MH112070. Dr C.H.Y. Fu acknowledged support from MRC grant G0802594.

REFERENCES

1. Kessler RC, Bromet EJ. The epidemiology of depression across cultures. Annu Rev Public Health 2013;34(1):119–38.
2. Whiteford HA, Degenhardt L, Rehm J, et al. Global burden of disease attributable to mental and substance use disorders: findings from the Global Burden of Disease Study 2010. Lancet 2013; 382(9904):1575–86.
3. American Psychiatric Association. Diagnostic and statistical manual of mental disorders. 5th edition 2013. Available at: https://dsm.psychiatryonline.org/doi/book/10.1176/appi.books.9781585624836. Accessed April 10, 2019.
4. World Health Organization, editor. International statistical classification of diseases and related health problems. 10th revision, 2nd edition. Geneva (Switzerland): World Health Organization; 2004.
5. Rush AJ, Trivedi MH, Wisniewski SR, et al. Acute and longer-term outcomes in depressed outpatients requiring one or several treatment steps: a STAR*D report. Am J Psychiatry 2006;163(11):1905–17.
6. Eaton WW, Shao H, Nestadt G, et al. Population-based study of first onset and chronicity in major depressive disorder. Arch Gen Psychiatry 2008; 65(5):513.
7. Major Depressive Disorder Working Group of the Psychiatric GWAS Consortium. A mega-analysis of genome-wide association studies for major depressive disorder. Mol Psychiatry 2013;18(4): 497–511.
8. Howard DM, Adams MJ, Clarke T-K, et al. Genome-wide meta-analysis of depression identifies 102 independent variants and highlights the importance of the prefrontal brain regions. Nat Neurosci 2019; 22(3):343–52.
9. Andersson E, Crowley JJ, Lindefors N, et al. Genetics of response to cognitive behavior therapy in adults with major depression: a preliminary report. Mol Psychiatry 2019;24(4):484–90.
10. Wigmore EM, Hafferty JD, Hall LS, et al. Genome-wide association study of antidepressant treatment resistance in a population-based cohort using health service prescription data and meta-analysis with GENDEP. Pharmacogenomics J 2019. https://doi.org/10.1038/s41397-019-0067-3.

11. Papez JW. A proposed mechanism of emotion. Arch Neur Psych 1937;38(4):725–43.

12. Aggleton JP, Brown MW. Episodic memory, amnesia, and the hippocampal-anterior thalamic axis. Behav Brain Sci 1999;22(3):425–44 [discussion: 444–89].

13. Maclean PD. Some psychiatric implications of physiological studies on frontotemporal portion of limbic system (visceral brain). Electroencephalogr Clin Neurophysiol 1952;4(4):407–18.

14. Heimer L, Van Hoesen GW. The limbic lobe and its output channels: implications for emotional functions and adaptive behavior. Neurosci Biobehav Rev 2006;30(2):126–47.

15. Schmaal L, Hibar DP, Sämann PG, et al. Cortical abnormalities in adults and adolescents with major depression based on brain scans from 20 cohorts worldwide in the ENIGMA Major Depressive Disorder Working Group. Mol Psychiatry 2017;22(6): 900–9.

16. Atkinson L, Sankar A, Adams TM, et al. Recent advances in neuroimaging of mood disorders: structural and functional neural correlates of depression, changes with therapy, and potential for clinical biomarkers. Curr Treat Options Psychiatry 2014;1(3): 278–93.

17. Arnone D, Job D, Selvaraj S, et al. Computational meta-analysis of statistical parametric maps in major depression: computational meta-analysis of parametric maps in major depression. Hum Brain Mapp 2016;37(4):1393–404.

18. Schmaal L, Veltman DJ, van Erp TGM, et al. Subcortical brain alterations in major depressive disorder: findings from the ENIGMA Major Depressive Disorder working group. Mol Psychiatry 2016; 21(6):806–12.

19. Wise T, Radua J, Via E, et al. Common and distinct patterns of grey-matter volume alteration in major depression and bipolar disorder: evidence from voxel-based meta-analysis. Mol Psychiatry 2017; 22(10):1455–63.

20. Cole J, Costafreda SG, McGuffin P, et al. Hippocampal atrophy in first episode depression: a meta-analysis of magnetic resonance imaging studies. J Affect Disord 2011;134(1–3):483–7.

21. Wang W, Zhao Y, Hu X, et al. Conjoint and dissociated structural and functional abnormalities in first-episode drug-naive patients with major depressive disorder: a multimodal meta-analysis. Sci Rep 2017;7(1):10401.

22. Boldrini M, Santiago AN, Hen R, et al. Hippocampal granule neuron number and dentate gyrus volume in antidepressant-treated and untreated major depression. Neuropsychopharmacology 2013;38(6): 1068–77.

23. Rajkowska G, Miguel-Hidalgo JJ, Wei J, et al. Morphometric evidence for neuronal and glial prefrontal cell pathology in major depression. Biol Psychiatry 1999;45(9):1085–98.

24. Ongür D, Drevets WC, Price JL. Glial reduction in the subgenual prefrontal cortex in mood disorders. Proc Natl Acad Sci U S A 1998;95(22): 13290–5.

25. Panizzon MS, Fennema-Notestine C, Eyler LT, et al. Distinct genetic influences on cortical surface area and cortical thickness. Cereb Cortex 2009;19(11): 2728–35.

26. Im K, Lee J-M, Lyttelton O, et al. Brain size and cortical structure in the adult human brain. Cereb Cortex 2008;18(9):2181–91.

27. Tang Y, Wang F, Xie G, et al. Reduced ventral anterior cingulate and amygdala volumes in medication-naïve females with major depressive disorder: a voxel-based morphometric magnetic resonance imaging study. Psychiatry Res 2007; 156(1):83–6.

28. Yucel K, McKinnon MC, Chahal R, et al. Anterior cingulate volumes in never-treated patients with major depressive disorder. Neuropsychopharmacol 2008;33(13):3157–63.

29. Hamilton JP, Siemer M, Gotlib IH. Amygdala volume in major depressive disorder: a meta-analysis of magnetic resonance imaging studies. Mol Psychiatry 2008;13(11):993–1000.

30. Paus T. Primate anterior cingulate cortex: where motor control, drive and cognition interface. Nat Rev Neurosci 2001;2(6):417–24.

31. Banks SJ, Eddy KT, Angstadt M, et al. Amygdala-frontal connectivity during emotion regulation. Soc Cogn Affect Neurosci 2007;2(4):303–12.

32. Costafreda SG, McCann P, Saker P, et al. Modulation of amygdala response and connectivity in depression by serotonin transporter polymorphism and diagnosis. J Affect Disord 2013;150(1):96–103.

33. Sheline YI, Wang PW, Gado MH, et al. Hippocampal atrophy in recurrent major depression. Proc Natl Acad Sci U S A 1996;93(9):3908–13.

34. Sheline YI, Sanghavi M, Mintun MA, et al. Depression duration but not age predicts hippocampal volume loss in medically healthy women with recurrent major depression. J Neurosci 1999;19(12):5034–43.

35. MacQueen GM, Campbell S, McEwen BS, et al. Course of illness, hippocampal function, and hippocampal volume in major depression. Proc Natl Acad Sci U S A 2003;100(3):1387–92.

36. Chen MC, Hamilton JP, Gotlib IH. Decreased hippocampal volume in healthy girls at risk of depression. Arch Gen Psychiatry 2010;67(3):270.

37. MacMaster FP, Kusumakar V. Hippocampal volume in early onset depression. BMC Med 2004;2(1):2.

38. Whittle S, Lichter R, Dennison M, et al. Structural brain development and depression onset during adolescence: a prospective longitudinal study. Am J Psychiatry 2014;171(5):564–71.

39. Pujol N, Penadés R, Junqué C, et al. Hippocampal abnormalities and age in chronic schizophrenia: morphometric study across the adult lifespan. Br J Psychiatry 2014;205(5):369–75.

40. Han K-M, Kim A, Kang W, et al. Hippocampal subfield volumes in major depressive disorder and bipolar disorder. Eur Psychiatry 2019;57:70–7.

41. Narr KL, Thompson PM, Szeszko P, et al. Regional specificity of hippocampal volume reductions in first-episode schizophrenia. Neuroimage 2004; 21(4):1563–75.

42. Treadway MT, Waskom ML, Dillon DG, et al. Illness progression, recent stress, and morphometry of hippocampal subfields and medial prefrontal cortex in major depression. Biol Psychiatry 2015; 77(3):285–94.

43. Cao B, Passos IC, Mwangi B, et al. Hippocampal subfield volumes in mood disorders. Mol Psychiatry 2017;22(9):1352–8.

44. Haukvik UK, Westlye LT, Mørch-Johnsen L, et al. In vivo hippocampal subfield volumes in schizophrenia and bipolar disorder. Biol Psychiatry 2015; 77(6):581–8.

45. Cole J, Toga AW, Hojatkashani C, et al. Subregional hippocampal deformations in major depressive disorder. J Affect Disord 2010;126(1–2):272–7.

46. Doolin K, Allers KA, Pleiner S, et al. Altered tryptophan catabolite concentrations in major depressive disorder and associated changes in hippocampal subfield volumes. Psychoneuroendocrinology 2018;95:8–17.

47. Ballmaier M, Narr KL, Toga AW, et al. Hippocampal morphology and distinguishing late-onset from early-onset elderly depression. Am J Psychiatry 2008;165(2):229–37.

48. Fu CHY, Costafreda SG. Neuroimaging-based biomarkers in psychiatry: clinical opportunities of a paradigm shift. Can J Psychiatry 2013;58(9):499–508.

49. Grosse L, Ambrée O, Jörgens S, et al. Cytokine levels in major depression are related to childhood trauma but not to recent stressors. Psychoneuroendocrinology 2016;73:24–31.

50. Danese A, Moffitt TE, Pariante CM, et al. Elevated inflammation levels in depressed adults with a history of childhood maltreatment. Arch Gen Psychiatry 2008;65(4):409–15.

51. McEwen BS. Stress and hippocampal plasticity. Annu Rev Neurosci 1999;22(1):105–22.

52. Herman JP. Regulation of adrenocorticosteroid receptor mRNA expression in the central nervous system. Cell Mol Neurobiol 1993;13(4):349–72.

53. Radley JJ, Arias CM, Sawchenko PE. Regional differentiation of the medial prefrontal cortex in regulating adaptive responses to acute emotional stress. J Neurosci 2006;26(50):12967–76.

54. Tavares RF, Corrêa FMA, Resstel LBM. Opposite role of infralimbic and prelimbic cortex in the tachycardiac response evoked by acute restraint stress in rats. J Neurosci Res 2009;87(11):2601–7.

55. Critchley HD, Mathias CJ, Josephs O, et al. Human cingulate cortex and autonomic control: converging neuroimaging and clinical evidence. Brain 2003; 126(10):2139–52.

56. Radley JJ, Williams B, Sawchenko PE. Noradrenergic innervation of the dorsal medial prefrontal cortex modulates hypothalamo-pituitary-adrenal responses to acute emotional stress. J Neurosci 2008;28(22): 5806–16.

57. Fu CHY, Reed LJ, Meyer JH, et al. Noradrenergic dysfunction in the prefrontal cortex in depression: an [15O] H2O PET study of the neuromodulatory effects of clonidine. Biol Psychiatry 2001;49(4): 317–25.

58. Cowen PJ, Browning M. What has serotonin to do with depression? World Psychiatry 2015;14(2): 158–60.

59. Rajkowska G, Mahajan G, Legutko B, et al. Length of axons expressing the serotonin transporter in orbitofrontal cortex is lower with age in depression. Neuroscience 2017;359:30–9.

60. Veerakumar A, Challis C, Gupta P, et al. Antidepressant-like effects of cortical deep brain stimulation coincide with pro-neuroplastic adaptations of serotonin systems. Biol Psychiatry 2014;76(3):203–12.

61. Arnone D, McKie S, Elliott R, et al. State-dependent changes in hippocampal grey matter in depression. Mol Psychiatry 2013;18(12):1265–72.

62. Fu CH, Costafreda SG, Sankar A, et al. Multimodal functional and structural neuroimaging investigation of major depressive disorder following treatment with duloxetine. BMC Psychiatry 2015;15(1):82.

63. Bartlett EA, DeLorenzo C, Sharma P, et al. Pretreatment and early-treatment cortical thickness is associated with SSRI treatment response in major depressive disorder. Neuropsychopharmacology 2018;43(11):2221–30.

64. Ohira K, Takeuchi R, Shoji H, et al. Fluoxetine-induced cortical adult neurogenesis. Neuropsychopharmacol 2013;38(6):909–20.

65. Frodl TS, Koutsouleris N, Bottlender R, et al. Depression-related variation in brain morphology over 3 years: effects of stress? Arch Gen Psychiatry 2008; 65(10):1156.

66. Roddy DW, Farrell C, Doolin K, et al. The hippocampus in depression: more than the sum of its parts? Advanced hippocampal substructure segmentation in depression. Biol Psychiatry 2019; 85(6):487–97.

67. Vythilingam M, Heim C, Newport J, et al. Childhood trauma associated with smaller hippocampal volume in women with major depression. Am J Psychiatry 2002;159(12):2072–80.

68. Infurna MR, Reichl C, Parzer P, et al. Associations between depression and specific childhood

experiences of abuse and neglect: a meta-analysis. J Affect Disord 2016;190:47–55.

69. Teasdale JD. Negative thinking in depression: cause, effect, or reciprocal relationship? Adv Behav Res Ther 1983;5(1):3–25.

70. Watkins PC, Vache K, Verney SP, et al. Unconscious mood-congruent memory bias in depression. J Abnorm Psychol 1996;105(1):34–41.

71. Groenewold NA, Opmeer EM, de Jonge P, et al. Emotional valence modulates brain functional abnormalities in depression: evidence from a meta-analysis of fMRI studies. Neurosci Biobehav Rev 2013;37(2):152–63.

72. Mayberg HS. Limbic-cortical dysregulation: a proposed model of depression. J Neuropsychiatry Clin Neurosci 1997;9(3):471–81.

73. Phillips ML, Drevets WC, Rauch SL, et al. Neurobiology of emotion perception II: implications for major psychiatric disorders. Biol Psychiatry 2003;54(5):515–28.

74. Arnone D. Functional MRI findings, pharmacological treatment in major depression and clinical response. Prog Neuropsychopharmacol Biol Psychiatry 2019;91:28–37.

75. Fu CHY, Williams SCR, Cleare AJ, et al. Attenuation of the neural response to sad faces in major depression by antidepressant treatment: a prospective, event-related functional magnetic resonance imaging study. Arch Gen Psychiatry 2004;61(9):877.

76. Arnone D, McKie S, Elliott R, et al. Increased amygdala responses to sad but not fearful faces in major depression: relation to mood state and pharmacological treatment. Am J Psychiatry 2012;169(8):841–50.

77. Fu CHY, Williams SCR, Cleare AJ, et al. Neural responses to sad facial expressions in major depression following cognitive behavioral therapy. Biol Psychiatry 2008;64(6):505–12.

78. Sankar A, Melin A, Lorenzetti V, et al. A systematic review and meta-analysis of the neural correlates of psychological therapies in major depression. Psychiatry Res Neuroimaging 2018;279:31–9.

79. Etkin A, Egner T, Kalisch R. Emotional processing in anterior cingulate and medial prefrontal cortex. Trends Cogn Sci 2011;15(2):85–93.

80. Gotlib IH, Joormann J. Cognition and depression: current status and future directions. Annu Rev Clin Psychol 2010;6:285–312.

81. Fu CHY, Steiner H, Costafreda SG. Predictive neural biomarkers of clinical response in depression: a meta-analysis of functional and structural neuroimaging studies of pharmacological and psychological therapies. Neurobiol Dis 2013;52:75–83.

82. Marwood L, Wise T, Perkins AM, et al. Meta-analyses of the neural mechanisms and predictors of response to psychotherapy in depression and anxiety. Neurosci Biobehav Rev 2018;95:61–72.

83. Costafreda SG, Brammer MJ, David AS, et al. Predictors of amygdala activation during the processing of emotional stimuli: a meta-analysis of 385 PET and fMRI studies. Brain Res Rev 2008;58(1):57–70.

84. Nouretdinov I, Costafreda SG, Gammerman A, et al. Machine learning classification with confidence: application of transductive conformal predictors to MRI-based diagnostic and prognostic markers in depression. Neuroimage 2011;56(2):809–13.

85. Fu CHY, Mourao-Miranda J, Costafreda SG, et al. Pattern classification of sad facial processing: toward the development of neurobiological markers in depression. Biol Psychiatry 2008;63(7):656–62.

86. Sankar A, Zhang T, Gaonkar B, et al. Diagnostic potential of structural neuroimaging for depression from a multi-ethnic community sample. Br J Psych Open 2016;2(04):247–54.

87. Drysdale AT, Grosenick L, Downar J, et al. Resting-state connectivity biomarkers define neurophysiological subtypes of depression. Nat Med 2017;23(1):28–38.

88. Kim HJ, Park J-Y, Seo SW, et al. Cortical atrophy pattern-based subtyping predicts prognosis of amnestic MCI: an individual-level analysis. Neurobiol Aging 2019;74:38–45.

89. Koutsouleris N, Meisenzahl EM, Borgwardt S, et al. Individualized differential diagnosis of schizophrenia and mood disorders using neuroanatomical biomarkers. Brain 2015;138(7):2059–73.

90. Dong A, Honnorat N, Gaonkar B, et al. CHIMERA: clustering of heterogeneous disease effects via distribution matching of imaging patterns. IEEE Trans Med Imaging 2016;35(2):612–21.

91. Varol E, Sotiras A, Davatzikos C, Alzheimer's Disease Neuroimaging Initiative. HYDRA: revealing heterogeneity of imaging and genetic patterns through a multiple max-margin discriminative analysis framework. Neuroimage 2017;145(Pt B):346–64.

92. Dong A, Toledo JB, Honnorat N, et al. Heterogeneity of neuroanatomical patterns in prodromal Alzheimer's disease: links to cognition, progression and biomarkers. Brain 2017;140(3):735–47.

93. Davatzikos C. Quantifying anatomical and functional heterogeneity in big datasets, using machine learning methods towards a dimensional neuroimaging framework. Biol Psychiatry 2018;83(9):S14–5.

94. Kaczkurkin AN, Sotiras A, Baller EB, et al. Neurostructural heterogeneity in youth with internalizing symptoms. Neuroscience 2019. https://doi.org/10.1101/614438.

95. Danhong W, Meiling L, Meiyun W, et al. Individual-specific functional connectivity markers track

dimensional and categorical features of psychotic illness. Mol Psychiatry 2018. https://doi.org/10.1038/s41380-018-0276-1.

96. Huang X, Gong Q, Sweeney JA, et al. Progress in psychoradiology, the clinical application of psychiatric neuroimaging. Br J Radiol 2019;92(1101):20181000.

97. Port JD. Diagnosis of attention deficit hyperactivity disorder by using MR imaging and radiomics: a potential tool for clinicians. Radiology 2018;287:631–2.

98. Sun H, Chen Y, Huang Q, et al. Psychoradiologic utility of MR imaging for diagnosis of attention deficit hyperactivity disorder: a radiomics analysis. Radiology 2018;287(2):620–30.

The Neurodevelopment of Autism from Infancy Through Toddlerhood

Jessica B. Girault, PhD*, Joseph Piven, MD

KEYWORDS

- Neurodevelopment • Neuroimaging • Psychoradiology • Infant • Brain • Autism spectrum disorder
- MR imaging • Diffusion tensor imaging

KEY POINTS

- Neuroimaging has played a key role in revealing brain phenotypes associated with autism spectrum disorder (ASD) during infancy and toddlerhood.
- A wealth of studies converge on several key findings, including brain overgrowth, increased extra-axial cerebrospinal fluid volume, altered white matter development, and aberrant structural and functional connectivity patterns in ASD.
- It is likely that ASD arises from multiple prenatal and postnatal pathogenic mechanisms involving neural proliferation and migration, synaptogenesis, pruning, myelination, and axonal development and connectivity.
- Predicting diagnostic and dimensional outcomes using neuroimaging data in infancy holds great promise for advancing clinical practice.
- Future work should focus on parsing heterogeneity in ASD, linking genetic variation to brain imaging data in infancy, charting the co-occurrence of developmental brain and behavior phenotypes, and coupling neuroimaging studies with basic science research.

INTRODUCTION

Autism spectrum disorder (ASD) is a neurodevelopmental disorder diagnosed in 1 in 59 children in the United States.[1] ASD is characterized by heterogeneous symptom profiles associated with varying levels of severity in social communication deficits and restricted and repetitive behaviors. There has been considerable interest in understanding the neurobiology of ASD, with neuroimaging playing a key role in describing the neuroanatomy and physiology of individuals with ASD for more than 3 decades. However, the vast majority of studies to date have occurred after diagnosis and been cross-sectional in nature,

collapsing across wide age ranges. Given that we now understand that brain development, and the development of ASD,[2–5] is nonlinear and dynamic, it is no surprise that nonreplication left the field with few tenable brain phenotypes in ASD and even less insight into pathogenesis.

An increased understanding of the heritable nature of the disorder and recurrence risk in families[6] led to a paradigm shift with the advent of the infant-sibling study design. Researchers began to follow the younger, high-risk siblings of older children with ASD, 20% of whom develop ASD themselves,[7] through infancy and into toddlerhood, providing a window into the period when ASD first emerges.[8,9] These prospective studies have

Disclosure Statement: J.B. Girault is funded by NIH T32-HD040127 to J. Piven. J. Piven is funded by NIH R01-HD055741, R01-MH118362, and U54-HD079124.
Carolina Institute for Developmental Disabilities, The University of North Carolina at Chapel Hill School of Medicine, 101 Renee Lynne Court, Chapel Hill, NC 27599, USA
* Corresponding author.
E-mail address: jbgirault@unc.edu

revealed that the diagnostic symptoms of ASD emerge during the latter part of the first and second year of life.[10–14] Differences in other developmental domains that are not necessarily specific to ASD, however, are detectable in the first year of life, including motor skills,[15–17] attention to faces and social scenes,[18–20] response to name,[21] visual reception,[15] and visual orienting.[22] Early in the second year of life, differences in language skills[9,15,23] and disengagement of visual attention[24] are also evident.

These behaviors arise during a highly dynamic period of postnatal brain growth,[25,26] marked by cortical expansion,[27,28] fiber myelination and maturation,[29,30] and functional organization of neural circuitry.[31,32] Infant-sibling studies incorporating neuroimaging have provided great insight into brain development in ASD, revealing that atypical brain phenotypes emerge during infancy, with altered developmental trajectories preceding the consolidation of symptoms that begins in the second year of life.[2] This body of work has enhanced our understanding of the developmental time course of early ASD, and recently demonstrated the possibility of using presymptomatic MR imaging in infants to predict diagnostic outcomes in toddlerhood,[33,34] an advancement with important implications for clinical practice.

In this article, we review neuroimaging studies of early ASD including structural, diffusion, and functional MR imaging from the early postnatal period through preschool. This review aims to synthesize information across studies to identify biomarkers endorsed across samples, outline the developmental time course of the emergence of ASD-related neural phenotypes, and identify candidate biological mechanisms. In addition, we outline recent studies using neural phenotypes and machine learning approaches to predict subsequent diagnosis and discuss the implications for clinical practice. This review concludes with future directions for the field, including the need to identify individual-specific areas of developmental concern, parse etiologic heterogeneity using neurologic features, incorporate indices of genetic variation into neuroimaging studies of early brain development, chart the co-occurrence of developmental brain and behavioral phenotypes in individuals, and continue to bridge in vivo MR imaging with basic science to reveal mechanistic insights into the pathophysiology of ASD.

STRUCTURAL MR IMAGING
Brain Overgrowth

Brain overgrowth in ASD has been widely documented, dating to the first reports of the phenomenon using MR imaging in adolescents and adults with ASD more than 2 decades ago.[35–37] These findings were later extended to young children,[38–46] with convergent evidence across studies suggesting that brain overgrowth was present by 2 years of age in children with ASD. Indirect evidence from head circumference measurements at birth and MR imaging in infancy and toddlerhood suggested that brain overgrowth was not present at birth, but emerged in the later part of the first year of life.[41] This finding was later confirmed using MR imaging in a cohort of 55 infants longitudinally examined from 6 to 24 months of age,[47] such that infants who developed ASD (n = 10) demonstrated faster rates of total brain volume growth resulting in increased brain volumes by 12 to 24 months of age compared with infants who did not develop ASD. A more recent, large-scale study (106 high-risk infants, 42 controls) has provided additional evidence for brain volume overgrowth between 12 and 24 months, and linked the rate of change in total brain volume during the second year of life to the severity of ASD-related social deficits.[33] Importantly, the investigators decomposed cortical volume into cortical thickness and surface area to reveal that faster rates of cortical surface area growth from 6 to 12 months of age precedes brain overgrowth in the second year of life in infants who later developed ASD (n = 15).[33] The rate of surface area expansion from 6 to 12 months was also correlated with total brain volume at 24 months of age. These findings directly support the hypothesis generated from prior work that cortical hyperexpansion drives brain overgrowth in ASD.[44] A machine learning approach to diagnostic classification using MR imaging measures at 6 and 12 months was also used in this study,[33] and is discussed in detail as follows.

Cortical Surface Area, Thickness, and Gyrification

The surface area and thickness of the cortex have been differentially examined, as opposed to jointly examined in studies of cortical volume, in only a handful of studies of young children with ASD. In the first study of its kind, Hazlett and colleagues[44] reported increases in the surface area of the frontal, temporal, and parietal lobes in 2-year-olds with ASD, findings that were replicated in a sample of 3-year-old boys with ASD.[48] A more recent study demonstrated both accelerated rates of total cortical surface area expansion, and regionalized expansion in areas in the occipital, temporal, and frontal lobes in infants who later went on to develop ASD, with robust rates of expansion notable in the visual cortex.[33] Taken together, these findings support the pathologic hyperexpansion of cortical surface area in ASD, with Hazlett and colleagues[33] tracing its origins to the first year of life. Each of these studies[33,44,48] found no evidence of differences in cortical thickness between infants and toddlers with ASD and controls. One study in 2-year-old to 5-year-old boys stands in contrast, reporting no differences in surface area but increased thickness in some localized cortical areas[49]; this may be due to the relatively small sample size (66 ASD, 29 controls) given a wider developmental age range, use of vertex-based image analysis pipelines (not used by the other 3 studies), or lack of detection of a brain overgrowth phenotype in their sample. Cortical thickness differences have been observed in adolescents and adults with ASD, although the direction of effect varies.[50–52] By using a mixed cross-sectional and longitudinal design including individuals with ASD and controls (ages 3–39 years), Zielinski and colleagues[53] provided some clarity to these incongruent findings. The investigators reported greater cortical thickness across multiple brain regions in childhood, followed by a crossing of trajectories in middle childhood and finally reduced regional cortical thickness in early adulthood in individuals with ASD.[53,54] In light of reports in infants and toddlers, it is likely that aberrant patterns of cortical thickness in ASD emerge sometime after age 3 and follow a dynamic developmental pattern thereafter. Cortical gyrification patterns, which may reflect surface area expansion, in young children with ASD are largely unknown. One recent study in boys (105 with ASD, 49 controls) ages 3 to 5 years found that at age 3, boys with ASD had reduced gyrification in the fusiform gyrus.[55] A longitudinal examination revealed that local indices of gyrification in boys with ASD increased across the preschool period in regions in the temporal, frontal, and parietal lobes,[55] whereas local gyrification was generally stable or decreasing in typically developing controls. This is consistent with other studies reporting increased gyrification in older children and adults with ASD.[56–60] Further studies in young children and infants will be needed to discern developmental gyrification patterns in early ASD.

Subcortical Structures

There has been considerable interest in the role of the amygdala, as a core region in the social brain, in the pathophysiology of ASD,[61] yet there have been relatively few studies exploring the development of the amygdala and other subcortical brain regions in early ASD. Sparks and colleagues[39]

found evidence of bilateral enlargement of the amygdala and hippocampus using MR imaging in a sample of 3-year-olds to 4-year-olds with ASD, although after adjusting for total brain volume, only amygdala volumes in a subset of children with more severe ASD remained significantly enlarged. A longitudinal follow-up of this cohort revealed that greater volumes in the right amygdala in toddlerhood related to poorer social and communication outcomes at age 6.[62] Similar findings were reported in another study of toddlers with ASD,[63] where increased amygdala size correlated with the severity of social and communication deficits, with a particularly robust amygdala phenotype reported in girls with ASD. In a longitudinal investigation of brain-behavior associations in toddlers with ASD (ages 2–4 years), Mosconi and colleagues[64] reported that amygdala enlargement was present and stable across the preschool period, but, in contrast to other earlier studies, found that increased amygdala volume conferred better joint attention among children with ASD. In a study of boys ages 18 to 42 months, several subcortical structures were found to have increased volume compared with typically developing controls including the amygdala (20% larger), caudate nucleus, globus pallidus, and putamen.[65] More recently, Qiu and colleagues[66] reported bilateral caudate enlargement from 2 to 4 years of age compared with children with developmental delay, and Pote and colleagues[67] reported an overall enlargement of subcortical regions in 4-month-old to 6-month-old infants at high familial risk for ASD (including infants who did and did not develop ASD, n = 26 total, n = 4 with ASD), with greater volumes associated with increased restricted and repetitive behaviors at 36 months. A study of infants at elevated familial risk for ASD found differential associations between amygdala, thalamus, and caudate volumes at age 1 and language abilities at age 2 in infants who were later diagnosed with ASD versus those with language delay only,[23] the investigators suggest this is reflective of distinct neural mechanisms, and likely genetic and environmental risk factors, governing language development in infants with ASD.

Cerebellum

Cerebellar structural abnormalities measured by MR imaging are frequently reported in older children and adults with ASD,[68,69] although the direction of effect varies.[69] Similar inconsistencies have been reported in studies of infants and toddlers. A study of 3-year-olds to 4-year-olds found that children with ASD fell between typically developing children (lowest cerebellar volumes) and children with developmental delays (greatest cerebellar volumes)[70]; the investigators explored associations between cerebellar volumes and child behavior and found no associations. Larger white matter volumes within the cerebellum in young children with ASD have also been reported,[40,42] as well as increased gray matter, although only in young girls.[42] Several other studies, however, found no differences in cerebellar volumes between cases and controls (ages 18 months to 5 years) after adjusting for total brain size.[39,41,44] Taken together, these finding suggest that cerebellar abnormalities may exist, but future work will be needed to arrive at a consensus in the literature. In addition, findings are highly dependent on statistical modeling, and studies should carefully control for overall brain size to ensure that findings of volumetric enlargement are specific to the cerebellum.

Corpus Callosum Morphology

The corpus callosum in older children, adolescents, and adults with ASD has been shown to be smaller in size when compared with controls.[71–73] Studies in young children ages 3 and older have found results consistent with these findings. A study in 3-year-olds to 4-year-olds found that midsagittal corpus callosum area was disproportionately small relative to total brain size in children with ASD compared with typically developing controls, with reduced area throughout the structure.[74] A more recent longitudinal study of 3-year-olds to 5-year-olds echoed these findings, reporting that children with ASD had smaller regions dedicated to fibers projecting to the superior frontal cortex compared with typically developing children.[75] In the only prospective study in infants, Wolff and colleagues[76] found that corpus callosum area and thickness were significantly greater at 6 and 12 months, but not 24 months, in infants with familial risk who went on to develop ASD, with the most prominent group differences found in the anterior region of the corpus callosum connecting the prefrontal cortex. This study also found that cross-sectional measures of area and thickness at 6 months of age were correlated with degree of restricted and repetitive behaviors at 24 months in infants who developed ASD. Taken together, these findings suggest that the development of the corpus callosum reflects a dynamic process whereby the size of the corpus callosum in individuals who develop ASD is increased compared with controls in the first year of life, normalizes by age 2, and becomes smaller sometime in the third year of life.

Increased Extra-Axial Cerebral Spinal Fluid Volume

Recent studies have detected increased volumes of extra-axial fluid, defined as the cerebrospinal fluid occupying the subarachnoid space surrounding the cortical surface of the brain, in the first year of life in infants who go on to develop ASD. In the original study to describe this phenomenon in early postnatal life, Shen and colleagues[47] prospectively assessed brain and behavioral development in a sample of 55 infants (33 at familial risk for ASD, 22 controls), reporting increases in extra-axial fluid volumes at 6 months that persisted through 24 months in infants who went on to develop ASD (n = 10). The investigators also reported that extra-axial fluid volumes at 6 months were related to ASD severity at the diagnostic visit. These findings were replicated in a much larger independent cohort of infants (n = 343, 221 at familial risk for ASD, 122 controls),[77] where those who went on to develop ASD (n = 47) had 18% more extra-axial fluid at 6 months when compared with controls. The investigators also reported that extra-axial fluid was disproportionately increased (25% greater than controls) in infants who went on to have the most severe ASD symptoms.[77] Shen and colleagues[78] extended these findings to a community-ascertained sample of 2-year-olds to 4-year-olds with ASD, reporting that increases in extra-axial fluid were nearly identical in children with ASD and familial risk and in children with ASD without familial risk, and persisted through age 3. The investigators also found that increased extra-axial fluid was associated with greater sleep problems and lower nonverbal ability in children with ASD. Taken together, these studies provide evidence that extra-axial fluid is a robust brain biomarker of ASD in early life that deserves further mechanistic study.

DIFFUSION MR IMAGING
White Matter Integrity and Connectivity

Using diffusion MR imaging, scientists have investigated white matter connectivity and integrity in ASD, although few studies have focused on the preschool period. In a small study of 7 children ages 1 to 3 years, Ben Bashat and colleagues[79] found children with ASD had greater fractional anisotropy (FA; reflects the degree of directed water diffusion in the brain, indicative of more mature white matter properties, including myelination, axonal density, and fiber packaging[80]) in the corpus callosum, corticospinal tract, and internal and external capsule when compared with typically developing children.

These early findings were in contrast to studies in adults that generally reported reduced FA in individuals with ASD,[81] but later supported by additional independent studies. Weinstein and colleagues[82] reported that children younger than 6 with ASD had increased FA in many fiber tracts compared with controls, including the cingulum, corpus callosum, and superior longitudinal fasciculus. Xiao and colleagues[46] reported similar findings, with increased FA in the corpus callosum, cingulum, and limbic system in toddlers with ASD. Another study reported increased FA in the frontal, temporal, and subcortical regions in young children with ASD (n = 32) compared with those with developmental delay (n = 16).[83] The investigators also reported an over-connectivity phenotype in ASD, although the methodology used uses direct streamline counts as a measure of connectivity strength, which has limitations.[84,85] Another more recent study of 97 toddlers (68 with ASD, 29 controls) found that FA in the corpus callosum fibers projecting to the temporal lobes were significantly greater in toddlers with ASD.[86] Two other studies found opposite patterns of FA in preschoolers with ASD versus controls. One cross-sectional study in 2-year-olds to 6-year-olds with ASD reported reduced FA in children with ASD compared with controls (including both typically developing children and children with developmental delay),[87] which is in contrast with other cross-sectional studies, possibly due to collapsing across a relatively wide age range. Another found lower FA in toddlers and children with ASD (mean age 5 years, ranging from 2 to 11 years), again possibly due to collapsing across a wide developmental range.[88]

Two longitudinal studies have provided clarity, revealing the dynamic developmental nature of white matter development in ASD. Wolff and colleagues[89] used an infant-sibling research design to prospectively follow 92 infants at familial risk for ASD at 6, 12, and 24 months of age. The investigators reported widespread significant differences in growth trajectories in major white matter fiber bundles in infants who went on to develop ASD (n = 28) compared with those who did not. Infants later diagnosed with ASD exhibited increased FA at 6 months of age followed by slower maturation through 24 months of age. In line with the study by Wolff and colleagues,[89] a study of 1-year-olds to 4-year-olds reported abnormal age-related changes in FA, with greater FA at younger ages and slower rates of change thereafter, especially in frontal fiber tracts.[90] Taken together, these findings suggest that ASD is characterized by increased FA in

the first year of life, marked by a slowing in maturation thereafter that may ultimately result in reduced FA values observed in older children and adults.

Newer methodological approaches have been used to consider white matter in the human brain as a network, or connectome.[91] Lewis and colleagues[92] estimated properties of white matter network efficiency in 2-year-olds and found that toddlers with ASD had reduced local and global efficiency, especially in sensory processing regions in the occipital and temporal lobes, compared with controls. In a follow-up study the investigators downward extended these findings to reveal deficits in white matter network efficiency as early as 6 months of age in infants who went on to develop ASD.[93]

There is a growing body of work linking white matter development and ASD-related behaviors in young children with ASD. Wolff and colleagues[94] recently reported that developmental changes in FA in cerebellar fibers and the corpus callosum in infants with ASD was positively associated with restricted and repetitive behaviors and response to sensory stimuli. Another study found that visual orienting at 7 months of age was associated with the microstructural organization of the splenium, but only in children without an ASD diagnosis, possibly suggesting an aberrant functional specialization of visual circuitry in ASD.[22] Lewis and colleagues[93] demonstrated the inefficiencies in white matter connectivity, especially in longitudinally in temporal regions, were associated with symptom severity at 24 months, findings echoed in a study by Fingher and colleagues[86] reporting that white matter integrity in the temporal segments of the corpus callosum in toddlers was associated with outcome measures of ASD severity at later ages. White matter correlates of language were studied in 104 preschool-aged boys with ASD,[95] and investigators reported that FA (and other measures of microstructure) in the bilateral inferior longitudinal fasciculus both differed within the ASD group based on level of language, and was associated with individual differences in language scores. In another recent study of language and white matter development, Liu and colleagues[96] reported altered lateralization patterns in language tracts in infants at familial risk for ASD (n = 16), with FA lateralization in 6-week-olds relating to language outcomes at 18 months and ASD symptomology at 36 months, although it is unclear how this relates to symptomology above the diagnostic threshold. These findings suggest that behavioral disruptions in ASD may result from a variety of alterations in white matter development that deserve further investigation.

FUNCTIONAL MR IMAGING
Auditory-Evoked Functional MR Imaging

Functional MR imaging (fMR imaging) studies assessing spontaneous fluctuations in blood oxygenation as an index of neural activity and connectivity in very young children with ASD were relatively sparse until recently. The first auditory-evoked fMR imaging study during natural sleep in young children with ASD found significant differences in brain activation in a distributed network in response to forward and backward speech stimuli,[97] with a rightward lateralization in speech perception networks in toddlers with ASD (n = 12). Using the same experimental approach, Eyler and colleagues[98] found that neural response to sound in infants ages 12 to 48 months later diagnosed with ASD (n = 40) was deficient in the left hemisphere and, again, abnormally right-lateralized in the temporal lobe compared with typically developing controls. In a follow-up study, Dinstein and colleagues[99] investigated spontaneous activity (by regressing out stimulus structure) to find that toddlers with ASD had significantly weaker interhemispheric synchronization in putative language areas including the inferior frontal gyrus. The strength of synchronization in the inferior frontal gyrus was positively correlated with verbal ability and negatively correlated with ASD severity. A more recent study by this group examining activation patterns found that toddlers with ASD who had poorer language performance a year later exhibited reduced activation in bilateral temporal and frontal brain regions when compared with controls.[100] Further, the investigators reported inverse and differential brain-behavior associations between the ASD groups and controls, suggesting aberrant functional specialization of language regions in ASD, in line with previous work.

Resting State Functional MR Imaging

In a study of whole-brain resting state functional connectivity, Chen and colleagues[101] revealed 2 atypical circuits in young children with ASD (n = 58, 29 with ASD, mean age 4.98 years, all children sedated): one composed of brain regions involved in social cognition exhibiting underconnectivity and the other composed of sensory-motor and visual brain regions showing overconnectivity in ASD. The investigators used support vector regression analysis to show that the 2 circuits were differentially related to, and predictive of, individual social deficits and restricted behaviors in their sample. Another study investigating social brain network function found that newborns with a family history of ASD (n = 18)

exhibited significantly greater neural activity in the right fusiform and left parietal cortex, and altered age-related changes in activity in the cingulate and insula,[102] although it is unclear whether these patterns are specific to the development of early ASD, as the diagnostic outcome of the infants was not reported. Weakened functional connectivity of the amygdala and several brain regions involved in social communication and repetitive behaviors has also been reported in young boys with ASD (mean age 3.5 years).[103] Repetitive behaviors and whole-brain functional connectivity was recently investigated in a study of infants at familial risk for ASD (n = 38).[104] The investigators found age-specific associations between functional connectivity in visual, control, and default mode networks, such that weaker positive correlations in activity at 12 months and between 12 and 24 months were associated with more restrictive and repetitive behaviors in infants at risk for ASD (n = 38, 20 went on to develop ASD). The direction of this association was reversed at age 2, such that more positive correlations between dorsal attention, subcortical, and default mode networks were associated with more restrictive and repetitive behaviors. The promise of resting state connectivity as an ASD biomarker was recently demonstrated, where functional connectivity features in 6-month-olds (derived from connections associated with ASD-relevant behaviors) were able to accurately predict diagnostic outcome at 24 months of age.[34] This study is described in detail as follows.

NEUROIMAGING FINDINGS IN A DEVELOPMENTAL CONTEXT

With growing evidence of brain changes in ASD preceding the emergence of the defining features of the disorder, it becomes critical to place these prodromal brain phenotypes in the context of early-emerging behaviors associated with ASD and ASD risk. Here we have developed a schematic (**Fig. 1**) demonstrating key findings from the neuroimaging literature reviewed above placed in a developmental context alongside behavioral and clinical phenotypes. Aberrant white matter development (indicated by FA[89] and corpus callosum size[76]) and increased extra-axial cerebrospinal fluid (CSF) volumes[47,77,78] are detectable by 6 months of age in infants who go on to develop ASD. This coincides with motor delays,[15–17] atypical visual orienting,[22] and aberrant attention to social stimuli.[18,20] It is important to note, however, that motor delays do not appear to be specific to children with ASD, and are also evident in

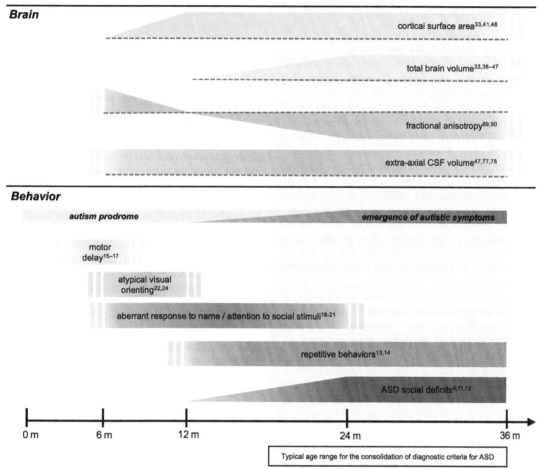

Fig. 1. Summary of neuroimaging findings in ASD in the context of emerging behaviors from infancy through toddlerhood. Brain changes in ASD precede the development of the defining diagnostic features of the disorder, and are temporally associated with behavioral changes in the first year of life that are both specific and nonspecific to ASD. Aberrant white matter integrity (FA) and increased extra-axial CSF volumes are detectable as early as 6 months of age in infants who go on to develop ASD, concurrent with motor and sensory delays. Surface area hyper-expansion in the first year of life precedes brain overgrowth in the second year, during which time ASD symptoms become apparent and begin to consolidate, while brain phenotypes remain relatively stable. Findings presented in the figure are those that are supported by multiple study paradigms (reference numbers noted in the figure), including at least one longitudinal study per phenotype. Double bars indicate that the start and/or end point of the trajectory is unknown or not well documented in the literature. Dashed lines in the top panel represent a reference to typical brain development, whereas bars above or below the dotted line indicate the brain phenotype is either increased or decreased relative to controls, respectively. For example, FA in ASD is increased at 6 months, not significantly different at 12 months, and decreased from 24 to 36 months when compared with controls. Repetitive behaviors and ASD social deficits are shown to continue past 36 months without citations, as these are diagnostic features that are, by definition, present in individuals with an ASD diagnosis.

high-risk infant siblings who do not meet diagnostic criteria.[16,105]

Surface area hyperexpansion in the first year of life precedes brain overgrowth in the second year.[33] Concurrently, infants who go on to develop ASD exhibit altered response to hearing their name beginning at 9 months and continuing through 24 months,[21] coinciding with differential trajectories in attention to eyes compared with controls,[19] and the emergence of ASD symptoms.[9,11–14] Taken together, these results begin to build a developmental timeline in which brain and behavioral phenotypes associated with ASD and ASD risk emerge during a prodromal period largely prior the second birthday, after which time diagnostic symptoms begin to consolidate.

CANDIDATE NEUROBIOLOGICAL MECHANISMS

The first 2 years of life are marked by rapid, dynamic brain growth, with total brain volume doubling in the first year,[106] largely driven by gray matter development, and specifically the expansion of cortical surface area.[27] In ASD, however, this postnatal developmental trajectory is disrupted. Findings from behavioral and neuroimaging studies of infants who go on to develop ASD suggest that the hyperexpansion of cortical surface area co-occurs with a prodromal period of motor, sensory, and visual orienting deficits observed from 6 to 12 months of age, followed by brain overgrowth and the emergence of autistic social deficits in the second year of life.[2] This highlights a central role for mechanisms governing surface area expansion in the pathophysiology of ASD.

The expansion of cortical surface area is thought to be governed by neural progenitor cell proliferation, differentiation, and migration,[107–110] with updated models specific to the gyrencephalic cortex pointing to the role of the fan-like expansion of outer radial glial (oRG) cells in tangential surface area growth.[108,109] The expansion of the oRG cell population is directly related to brain size,[107] as oRG give rise to highly proliferative intermediate progenitor cells that undergo amplifying divisions during neurogenesis.[111] Evidence for the potential role of neural progenitor proliferation and neurogenesis in the development of ASD has been supported by a wealth of preclinical, genetic, and postmortem data reviewed in detail elsewhere.[112] It is further supported by recent studies demonstrating that neural progenitor cells derived from individuals with ASD display excess proliferation compared with controls,[113,114] with the level of proliferation relating to the degree of brain overgrowth observed using MR imaging.[113] Another similarly designed study found evidence of significant developmental acceleration in neuronal differentiation in ASD, resulting in neurons with more complex branching.[115] Increased brain volume and macrocephaly are hallmarks of several genetically defined autistic syndromes including 16p11 deletion, Chd8 and PTEN mutations,[116–119] providing a window into the underlying pathophysiology in at least a subset of individuals with ASD.

There is evidence that the overproduction of neurons alters neural connectivity, with downstream consequences for circuit function and behavior. In mice, the induced overpopulation of upper-layer pyramidal neurons disrupts the development of dendrites and spines and alters the laminar distribution of neurons, resulting in dysregulated synaptic connectivity and autismlike behaviors.[120] This aligns with studies reporting alterations in synaptogenesis and neuronal excitability,[113] and relatively more inhibitory neurons and synapses in organoids derived from cells of patients with ASD with macrocephaly.[114] Another preclinical study observed postnatal brain overgrowth, altered long-range functional connectivity, motor delay, and anomalous response to social stimuli in Chd8 mutant mice, suggesting that altered brain growth and disrupted long-range wiring may underlie behavioral deficits observed in at least some subtypes of ASD.[121] Other evidence suggests that brain overgrowth in ASD may also be related to alterations in mechanisms governing synaptic pruning and the refinement of neural circuitry that occurs during early postnatal development.[122] Experience-dependent plasticity has particularly notable impacts on primary sensory systems,[123] which also exhibit surface area hyperexpansion in infants who go on to develop ASD.[33] Deficits in the cellular mechanisms controlling experience-dependent elimination of synapses, specifically long-term depression (LTD), has been observed in several mouse models of ASD and related neurodevelopmental disorders.[124–127] Further, locally-balanced excitation and inhibition play a key role in modulating competition between synapses and ultimately in defining the critical period for plasticity and refinement[123]; an imbalance in excitatory and inhibitory synapses like that reported by Marchetto and colleagues[113] in ASD-derived neuronal cultures could have marked impacts on the development of neural circuitry.

When considering brain overgrowth and behavioral findings together, a picture emerges of how ASD may develop in early life. Cortical hyperexpansion from 6 to 12 months, especially in the visual cortex,[33] may underlie concurrent deficits in visual orienting behaviors,[19,22] in turn altering experience-dependent neuronal development and ultimately resulting in inefficiently pruned circuits, brain overgrowth, and the emergence of ASD traits.[2] Although it is also possible that brain volume overgrowth is secondary to the increase in intermediate progenitor cells and less influenced by experience-dependent pruning mechanisms.

Neuroimaging findings of increased extra-axial fluid volumes implicate additional pathogenic mechanisms in ASD. A body of recent work has elucidated the role of cerebrospinal fluid (CSF) in brain development and function.[128] Lehtinen and colleagues[129] found that CSF contained growth factors with age-dependent effects on neuronal proliferation, suggesting an important role for CSF composition in cortical development. Further, increased volumes of extra-axial fluid suggest a disruption in the circulation of CSF and an accumulation of brain metabolites that impact brain function including amyloid beta and pro-inflammatory cytokines.[130,131] These findings, coupled with evidence that extra-axial fluid volume is increased *before* surface area hyperexpansion,[47,77] implicates the functional role of CSF in pathophysiology of ASD and related neurodevelopmental disorders. Preclinical work will be needed to further explore a potential regulatory role for CSF in surface area hyperexpansion in ASD.

Alterations in corpus callosum morphology and in the development of white matter microstructure in early ASD implicates processes governing myelination, axon caliber, density and axonal connectivity. A study of several mouse models of ASD recently identified a significant enrichment of myelination genes, and gene-set analysis implicated genes and pathways associated with myelination and oligodendrocyte differentiation.[132] Altered oligodendrocyte function has been documented in *Pten*-mutant mouse models of ASD, such that oligodendrocyte progenitor cells developed too early, resulting in reduced myelin sheaths,[133] which would impede information transfer along axons. The finding of reduced myelin sheath thickness has also been observed in postmortem studies of individuals with ASD.[134] This same study[134] also reported a decrease in large-diameter long-range axons and an increase in small-diameter short-range axons in the frontal cortex, consistent with inefficient connectivity observed in imaging studies in infants and toddlers with ASD.[92,93] White matter integrity and connectivity also may be altered through experience-dependent myelination,[135,136] in which oligodendrocytes selectively myelinate axons that receive more input from neurons, in line with altered excitability observed in neurons derived from patients with ASD.[113]

In summary, it is likely that ASD arises from multiple prenatal and postnatal pathogenic mechanisms involving neural proliferation and migration, synaptogenesis, pruning, myelination, and axonal development and connectivity, with each of these processes having important independent and interactive contributions to brain development. This is no surprise, as a large-scale genetic study of more than 18,000 individuals with ASD identified that one's risk for ASD depends on the level of polygenic burden of thousands of common variants in a dose-dependent manner.[137] Further, many of the genes implicated in ASD are pleiotropic in nature, impacting numerous cellular and molecular pathways.[138] This, coupled with what is known about the development of ASD

from neuroimaging studies, suggests an early-emerging vulnerability that is nonspecific in nature with effects on brain development detectable as early as the first year of life. This mechanistic complexity likely underlies the notable behavioral and clinical variability observed in ASD, calling for a need to parse phenotypic heterogeneity to arrive at more parsimonious etiologic models.

PREDICTING AUTISM SPECTRUM DISORDER DIAGNOSIS
Presymptomatic Prediction Using MR Imaging

Two recent studies using a prospective longitudinal design coupled with machine learning approaches demonstrated the potential for predicting ASD diagnosis at 24 months using infant MR imaging scans collected in the first year of life. Both studies followed younger siblings of older children with ASD from 6 months of age and collected MR imaging scans, behavioral measures, and clinical outcomes. In the first study, the investigators used supervised deep learning to build a classification algorithm that relied primarily on measures of regional cortical surface area growth from 6 to 12 months of age to predict ASD diagnostic outcome at 24 months.[33] This algorithm correctly predicted diagnosis in a sample of 106 infants at risk for ASD (15 received a diagnosis at 24 months) with 88% sensitivity, 95% specificity, and a positive predictive value (PPV) of 81%. This study is notable for 2 major reasons: (1) it significantly outperformed behavioral measures in the first 2 years in predicting diagnostic outcome,[139–142] and (2) it used features derived from a standard structural MR imaging *preceding* the onset of the defining behavioral features of the disorder, raising the possibility of assigning infants to presymptomatic intervention during a period of heightened neural plasticity. The other study from the same group found that a support vector regression machine using whole-brain functional connectivity matrices, culled to connections significantly correlated with 24-month scores on measures of social behavior, language, motor development, and repetitive behavior, could predict diagnostic outcome with 82% sensitivity, 100% specificity, and a PPV of 100% in a sample of 59 high-risk infants, 11 of whom received a diagnosis.[34] Both of these studies pave the way for larger-scale investigations of presymptomatic identification of illness risk using MR imaging.

Diagnostic Prediction with MR Imaging: Best Practices in an Emerging Field

Machine learning, and particularly deep learning, have recently taken on a prominent role in neuroimaging research by allowing for the design of powerful classifiers able to exploit complex relationships between brain structural and functional features and cognitive and clinical phenotypes.[143] Several supervised discriminative machine learning methods have gained popularity for use with MR imaging datasets, perhaps the most popular (especially in the context of low-dimensional and limited datasets), being support vector machines (SVM), followed by, more recently, deep learning (DL). Following a feature reduction step, SVM works by finding the optimal linear plane separating classes (ie, diagnostic groups) using the original data (linear SVM), or data mapped into a new feature space using pre-defined kernel functions (nonlinear SVM) where classes become linearly separable.[144] On the other hand, with the increasing availability of larger neuroimaging datasets, DL algorithms have shown success in automatically identifying the optimal data representation in a data-driven manner, bypassing the need for prior selection of an appropriate nonlinear mapping.[143] This distinction is evidenced in the studies discussed above, where Hazlett and colleagues[33] used a DL approach that did not require a separate feature reduction step before, or separate from, building the algorithm, whereas Emerson and colleagues[34] reduced their connectivity features to those correlated with behavior before building the SVM classifier. Potential advantages of DL methods over SVM include that input features are learned from the data and not derived, which is less prone to overfitting, and the ability of DL to achieve a higher level of abstraction and complexity, allowing for the detection of more subtle patterns in the data.[143] For further information on machine learning algorithms used in pediatric neuroimaging, see a recent review by Mostapha and Styner.[145] Regardless of the approach taken, these methods should be used with the oversight of an experienced artificial intelligence scientist, statistician, or an engineer who regularly applies machine learning algorithms to high-dimensional datasets. Equally importantly, insight from individuals with clinical knowledge of the disorder will be critical in interpreting the complex results generated from these types of models.

With regard to best practices for conducting neuroimaging-based prediction studies, several key topics emerge, including sample size and generalizability, interpretation, and methodological transparency. Sample size is a major factor in designing accurate, generalizable supervised classification algorithms, particularly when dealing with MR imaging datasets that are as heterogeneous as those observed in early postnatal

development.[145] Future work using large, publicly available datasets, with compatible MR imaging sequences, age windows, and serial scans, will help combat this problem, alongside using rigorous cross-validation methods to ensure that the trained models generalize to unseen data. Class-imbalance is another major issue in predicting outcomes with low prevalence in the population. Algorithms tend to optimally recognize classes (or outcomes) with larger training samples, as opposed to minority samples with fewer training samples,[145] as would be the case with predicting an ASD diagnosis. There are new methods on the rise for addressing these concerns, including synthetic oversampling strategies.[146,147] Once classification algorithms are built and tested, it is scientifically critical to understand which features derived from the MR images (ie, which brain connections or regions) contributed to the classification. At the moment, it is still challenging to interpret what DL models have learned, although methods to solve this problem are increasingly proposed,[145] including backtrack methods like the one used by Hazlett and colleagues.[33] Finally, to share knowledge and create standards for best practice in the field, transparency is needed in the reporting and sharing of machine learning algorithms used in publications. Investigators should outline the rationale for the selection of the machine learning algorithm used in the study and report sample sizes, cross-validation and training, and testing procedures. Steps taken to address class-imbalance and details regarding tuning and optimization parameters should also be noted. Finally, the steps taken to interpret the findings, including methods used for identifying information learned by the algorithm and clinically-relevant performance metrics (specificity, sensitivity, PPV) should be included. The code used for building algorithms and conducting analyses must be made readily available to others for verification and replication.

Clinical and Ethical Considerations

Presymptomatic, individualized prediction at the large scale has substantial implications for shaping clinical practice, yet it comes with ethical implications[148] that must be carefully considered. The transition from group-level correlations to individual-level prediction in neuroscience is a key step toward improving the lives of individuals, and begins with carefully replicating pioneering studies by applying their models to new, independent datasets.[149] The development of psychoradiology, however, has shown promise in this regard aiming to achieve the individualized prediction for psychiatric disorders,[150–154] The next step is to integrate validated algorithms into clinical practice, in keeping with the precision medicine framework designed to assign individuals to personal treatment plans, maximizing treatment efficacy.[155] Although there are some evidence-based behavioral interventions for early ASD,[156–159] preemptive intervention has yet to be proven successful.[160] This both highlights the urgent need for developing and testing presymptomatic interventions, and raises the concern of implementing early diagnostic screening if no validated treatment options are available. Neuroimaging should be harnessed as a biologically-based screening tool that may offer insights into when and how to intervene, guiding future research.

FUTURE DIRECTIONS
Predicting Dimensional Outcomes

A major next step for the field will be to develop methodologies to predict individualized areas of concern, as ASD and other neurodevelopmental disorders exhibit substantial phenotypic variability. In addition, more than one-quarter of infants at familial risk for ASD will develop subthreshold atypical behaviors in the first years of life,[105] and could also be candidates for targeted intervention. Neuroimaging studies using machine learning approaches have demonstrated the possibility of individualized prediction of cognitive outcomes in toddlerhood using neonatal diffusion MR imaging scans[161,162]; future work should consider applying similar methodologies to infants at risk for ASD. Using MR imaging to target intervention to the first year of life may be most beneficial, as behaviors appear to be more separable and potentially more targetable in infancy.[163]

Parsing Heterogeneity

ASD has a strong heritable component, but complex genetic origins that overlap with other neuropsychiatric disorders, calling for a need to move beyond the traditional clinical diagnostic model to one increasingly guided by biology.[164] However, although heterogeneity in brain functioning is observable in psychiatric disorders and across individuals,[165–168] it is rarely considered in experimental designs. Parsing heterogeneity in neurodevelopmental profiles is likely a promising avenue for improving our understanding of the diversity and variability in symptomology associated with complex neuropsychiatric disorders, and is a major focus of the National Institute of Mental Health Research Diagnostic Criteria (RDoC) project.[169] Novel approaches to implementing clustering algorithms to identify subgroups in the population based on neural features has great promise to reveal meaningful insight into both etiology and treatment. In a similar manner, a developmental approach should be taken to identify subgroups with similar trajectories of the disorder, likely to be reflective of distinct etiologies.[170]

Relating Autism Spectrum Disorder Genetic Liability to Neurodevelopment

Although significant advances in genetics have identified de novo mutations in a portion of the ASD population, common,[171,172] additive[171,173] polygenic variation is thought to account for the vast majority of ASD cases. It is currently unknown how heritable common background genetic variation and polygenic risk for ASD contribute to individual differences in brain development during infancy and toddlerhood. The familial nature of the infant-sibling study design is well suited to explore these associations. Recent work in syndromic ASD has demonstrated the predictive power of background genetic factors for behavioral development in young children,[174] and future studies should extend this to idiopathic ASD, using neuroimaging to reveal etiologic insights into the early behavioral manifestation of the disorder.

Identifying Developmental Associations Between Brain and Behavior Phenotypes

Infants who go on to develop ASD, *as a group*, exhibit a variety of brain phenotypes, including brain overgrowth, increased extra-axial fluid volumes, abnormal development of the corpus callosum and other white matter pathways, and altered functional brain connectivity patterns. None of these phenotypes, on their own, are sufficient to predict diagnosis or identify causal mechanisms, pointing to multiple etiologies both *within* and *between* individuals. To date, we do not have a clear understanding of how these brain phenotypes are related in individuals, or how they link to behavior. Some of the earliest behaviors disrupted in infants who go on to develop ASD include motor skills, which have notable implications for later-emerging language and communication abilities.[175–177] Charting the developmental co-emergence and co-occurrence of brain and behavioral phenotypes in ASD from infancy through diagnosis should be a major scientific goal in the next generation of infant-sibling studies. Such detailed phenotypic developmental mapping would greatly improve our understanding of the unfolding of ASD, possibly revealing distinct etiologic subgroups.

Linking MR Imaging and Basic Science

Recently, substantial strides in basic science have allowed for the use of neural stem cells to recapitulate in vivo brain development in vitro. Several reports reviewed here used cells derived from individuals with ASD and macrocephaly to mimic early prenatal cortical development.[113–115] These studies represent an important step for the field in relating brain phenotypes observed in MR imaging to in vitro models derived from the same individuals, although methodological advances will be needed to allow for modeling later stages of brain development[178] that may be more central to ASD.[2] Future work should move beyond only studying individuals with ASD and brain overgrowth phenotypes[113–115] to reveal broader insights into etiology.

SUMMARY

Brain phenotypes derived from neuroimaging provide the earliest distinction between infants at risk for ASD and typically developing children, with group differences noted during the pre-symptomatic period before aberrant behavior that are reliably detectable. A wealth of studies converge on several key findings including brain overgrowth, increased extra-axial fluid volumes, altered white matter development, and aberrant structural and functional connectivity patterns in individuals with ASD. This implicates a variety of neurobiological mechanisms that both independently and jointly contribute to brain and behavioral development in early childhood. The field has made significant strides in describing brain phenotypes in ASD, and has recently taken steps toward implementing individualized prediction models to identify infants at heightened risk for developing ASD, calling for an urgent need for the concurrent development of effective presymptomatic interventions. In the coming years, scientists will need to focus on a variety of key areas requiring further investigation, including tackling the problem of etiologic heterogeneity and linking brain and behavioral development to underlying genetic mechanisms, a goal that will be achieved through a multidisciplinary approach combining neuroimaging, behavioral, and basic science research.

ACKNOWLEDGMENTS

The authors thank Mahmoud Mostapha and Martin Styner for their scientific overview as experts in applying DL methods to infant neuroimaging datasets.

REFERENCES

1. Baio J, Wiggins L, Christensen DL, et al. Prevalence of autism spectrum disorder among children aged 8 years - autism and developmental disabilities monitoring network, 11 sites, United States, 2014. MMWR Surveill Summ 2018;67(6):1–23.
2. Piven J, Elison JT, Zylka MJ. Toward a conceptual framework for early brain and behavior development in autism. Mol Psychiatry 2017;22(10):1385–94.
3. Wolff JJ, Jacob S, Elison JT. The journey to autism: insights from neuroimaging studies of infants and toddlers. Dev Psychopathol 2018;30(2):479–95.
4. Wolff JJ, Piven J. On the emergence of autism: neuroimaging findings from birth to preschool. Neuropsychiatry 2013;3(2):209–22.
5. Swanson MR, Piven J. Neurodevelopment of autism: the first three years of life. In: Casanova MF, El-Baz A, Suri JS, editors. Autism imaging and devices. Boca Raton (FL): CRC Press; 2017. p. 37–57.
6. Szatmari P, Jones MB, Zwaigenbaum L, et al. Genetics of autism: overview and new directions. J Autism Dev Disord 1998;28(5):351–68.
7. Ozonoff S, Young GS, Carter A, et al. Recurrence risk for autism spectrum disorders: a Baby Siblings Research Consortium study. Pediatrics 2011; 128(3):e488–95.
8. Landa R, Garrett-Mayer E. Development in infants with autism spectrum disorders: a prospective study. J Child Psychol Psychiatry 2006;47(6): 629–38.
9. Zwaigenbaum L, Bryson S, Rogers T, et al. Behavioral manifestations of autism in the first year of life. Int J Dev Neurosci 2005;23(2–3):143–52.
10. Rogers SJ. What are infant siblings teaching us about autism in infancy? Autism Res 2009;2(3): 125–37.
11. Ozonoff S, Iosif A-M, Baguio F, et al. A prospective study of the emergence of early behavioral signs of autism. J Am Acad Child Adolesc Psychiatry 2010; 49(3):256–66.e1–2.
12. Landa RJ, Gross AL, Stuart EA, et al. Developmental trajectories in children with and without autism spectrum disorders: the first 3 years. Child Dev 2012;84(2):429–42.
13. Elison JT, Wolff JJ, Reznick JS, et al. Repetitive behavior in 12-month-olds later classified with autism spectrum disorder. J Am Acad Child Adolesc Psychiatry 2014;53(11):1216–24.
14. Wolff JJ, Botteron KN, Dager SR, et al. Longitudinal patterns of repetitive behavior in toddlers with autism. J Child Psychol Psychiatry 2014;55(8):945–53.
15. Estes A, Zwaigenbaum L, Gu H, et al. Behavioral, cognitive, and adaptive development in infants with autism spectrum disorder in the first 2 years of life. J Neurodev Disord 2015;7(1):24.

16. Iverson JM, Shic F, Wall CA, et al. Early motor abilities in infants at heightened versus low risk for ASD: a Baby Siblings Research Consortium (BSRC) study. J Abnorm Psychol 2019;128(1): 69–80.

17. Flanagan JE, Landa R, Bhat A, et al. Head lag in infants at risk for autism: a preliminary study. Am J Occup Ther 2012;66(5):577–85.

18. Chawarska K, Macari S, Shic F. Decreased spontaneous attention to social scenes in 6-month-old infants later diagnosed with autism spectrum disorders. Biol Psychiatry 2013;74(3):195–203.

19. Jones W, Klin A. Attention to eyes is present but in decline in 2–6-month-old infants later diagnosed with autism. Nature 2013;504(7480):427–31.

20. Shic F, Macari S, Chawarska K. Speech disturbs face scanning in 6-month-old infants who develop autism spectrum disorder. Biol Psychiatry 2014; 75(3):231–7.

21. Miller M, Iosif A-M, Hill M, et al. Response to name in infants developing autism spectrum disorder: a prospective study. J Pediatr 2017;183:141–6.e1.

22. Elison JT, Paterson SJ, Wolff JJ, et al. White matter microstructure and atypical visual orienting in 7-month-olds at risk for autism. Am J Psychiatry 2013;170(8):899–908.

23. Swanson MR, Shen MD, Wolff JJ, et al. Subcortical brain and behavior phenotypes differentiate infants with autism versus language delay. Biol Psychiatry Cogn Neurosci Neuroimaging 2017; 2(8):664–72.

24. Elsabbagh M, Fernandes J, Jane Webb S, et al. Disengagement of visual attention in infancy is associated with emerging autism in toddlerhood. Biol Psychiatry 2013;74(3):189–94.

25. Gilmore JH, Knickmeyer RC, Gao W. Imaging structural and functional brain development in early childhood. Nat Rev Neurosci 2018;19(3):123–37.

26. Bullins J, Jha SC, Knickmeyer RC, et al. Brain development during the preschool period. In: Luby J, editor. Handbook of preschool mental health. New York: Guilford Press; 2016. p. 73–97.

27. Lyall AE, Shi F, Geng X, et al. Dynamic development of regional cortical thickness and surface area in early childhood. Cereb Cortex 2015;25(8): 2204–12.

28. Li G, Wang L, Shi F, et al. Mapping longitudinal development of local cortical gyrification in infants from birth to 2 years of age. J Neurosci 2014; 34(12):4228–38.

29. Girault JB, Cornea E, Goldman BD, et al. White matter microstructural development and cognitive ability in the first 2 years of life. Hum Brain Mapp 2018;111(20):7456.

30. Geng X, Gouttard S, Sharma A, et al. Quantitative tract-based white matter development from birth to age 2 years. Neuroimage 2012;61(3):542–57.

31. Gao W, Alcauter S, Smith JK, et al. Development of human brain cortical network architecture during infancy. Brain Struct Funct 2015;220(2):1173–86.

32. Gao W, Lin W, Grewen K, et al. Functional connectivity of the infant human brain: plastic and modifiable. Neuroscientist 2016. https://doi.org/10.1177/1073858416635986.

33. Hazlett HC, Gu H, Munsell BC, et al. Early brain development in infants at high risk for autism spectrum disorder. Nature 2017;542(7641):348–51.

34. Emerson RW, Adams C, Nishino T, et al. Functional neuroimaging of high-risk 6-month-old infants predicts a diagnosis of autism at 24 months of age. Sci Transl Med 2017;9(393):eaag2882.

35. Piven J, Arndt S, Bailey J, et al. An MRI study of brain size in autism. Am J Psychiatry 1995;152(8): 1145–9.

36. Piven J, Arndt S, Bailey J, et al. Regional brain enlargement in autism: a magnetic resonance imaging study. J Am Acad Child Adolesc Psychiatry 1996;35(4):530–6.

37. Piven J, Nehme E, Simon J, et al. Magnetic resonance imaging in autism: measurement of the cerebellum, pons, and fourth ventricle. Biol Psychiatry 1992;31(5):491–504.

38. Courchesne E, Karns CM, Davis HR, et al. Unusual brain growth patterns in early life in patients with autistic disorder: an MRI study. Neurology 2001; 57(2):245–54.

39. Sparks BF, Friedman SD, Shaw DW, et al. Brain structural abnormalities in young children with autism spectrum disorder. Neurology 2002;59(2): 184–92.

40. Akshoomoff N, Lord C, Lincoln AJ, et al. Outcome classification of preschool children with autism spectrum disorders using MRI brain measures. J Am Acad Child Adolesc Psychiatry 2004;43(3): 349–57.

41. Hazlett HC, Poe M, Gerig G, et al. Magnetic resonance imaging and head circumference study of brain size in autism: birth through age 2 years. Arch Gen Psychiatry 2005;62(12):1366–76.

42. Bloss CS, Courchesne E. MRI neuroanatomy in young girls with autism: a preliminary study. J Am Acad Child Adolesc Psychiatry 2007;46(4):515–23.

43. Nordahl CW, Lange N, Li DD, et al. Brain enlargement is associated with regression in preschool-age boys with autism spectrum disorders. Proc Natl Acad Sci U S A 2011;108(50):20195–200.

44. Hazlett HC, Poe MD, Gerig G, et al. Early brain overgrowth in autism associated with an increase in cortical surface area before age 2 years. Arch Gen Psychiatry 2011;68(5):467–76.

45. Schumann CM, Bloss CS, Barnes CC, et al. Longitudinal magnetic resonance imaging study of cortical development through early childhood in autism. J Neurosci 2010;30(12):4419–27.

46. Xiao Z, Qiu T, Ke X, et al. Autism spectrum disorder as early neurodevelopmental disorder: evidence from the brain imaging abnormalities in 2-3 years old toddlers. J Autism Dev Disord 2014;44(7): 1633–40.

47. Shen MD, Nordahl CW, Young GS, et al. Early brain enlargement and elevated extra-axial fluid in infants who develop autism spectrum disorder. Brain 2013;136(Pt 9):2825–35.

48. Ohta H, Nordahl CW, Iosif A-M, et al. Increased surface area, but not cortical thickness, in a subset of young boys with autism spectrum disorder. Autism Res 2016;9(2):232–48.

49. Raznahan A, Lenroot R, Thurm A, et al. Mapping cortical anatomy in preschool aged children with autism using surface-based morphometry. Neuroimage Clin 2013;2:111–9.

50. Hardan AY, Muddasani S, Vemulapalli M, et al. An MRI study of increased cortical thickness in autism. Am J Psychiatry 2006;163(7):1290–2.

51. Hyde KL, Samson F, Evans AC, et al. Neuroanatomical differences in brain areas implicated in perceptual and other core features of autism revealed by cortical thickness analysis and voxel-based morphometry. Hum Brain Mapp 2010; 31(4):556–66.

52. Hadjikhani N, Joseph RM, Snyder J, et al. Anatomical differences in the mirror neuron system and social cognition network in autism. Cereb Cortex 2006;16(9):1276–82.

53. Zielinski BA, Prigge MBD, Nielsen JA, et al. Longitudinal changes in cortical thickness in autism and typical development. Brain 2014;137(Pt 6): 1799–812.

54. Wolff JJ, Piven J. Neurodevelopmental disorders: accelerating progress in autism through developmental research. Nat Rev Neurol 2014;10(8):431–2.

55. Libero LE, Schaer M, Li DD, et al. A longitudinal study of local gyrification index in young boys with autism spectrum disorder. Cereb Cortex 2018;33(6):2575–87.

56. Williams EL, El-Baz A, Nitzken M, et al. Spherical harmonic analysis of cortical complexity in autism and dyslexia. Transl Neurosci 2012;3(1):36–40.

57. Kohli JS, Kinnear MK, Fong CH, et al. Local cortical gyrification is increased in children with autism spectrum disorders, but decreases rapidly in adolescents. Cereb Cortex 2019;29(6):2412–23.

58. Hardan AY, Jou RJ, Keshavan MS, et al. Increased frontal cortical folding in autism: a preliminary MRI study. Psychiatry Res 2004;131(3):263–8.

59. Nordahl CW, Dierker D, Mostafavi I, et al. Cortical folding abnormalities in autism revealed by surface-based morphometry. J Neurosci 2007; 27(43):11725–35.

60. Shokouhi M, Williams JHG, Waiter GD, et al. Changes in the sulcal size associated with autism spectrum disorder revealed by sulcal morphometry. Autism Res 2012;5(4):245–52.

61. Baron-Cohen S, Ring HA, Bullmore ET, et al. The amygdala theory of autism. Neurosci Biobehav Rev 2000;24(3):355–64.

62. Munson J, Dawson G, Abbott R, et al. Amygdalar volume and behavioral development in autism. Arch Gen Psychiatry 2006;63(6):686.

63. Schumann CM, Barnes CC, Lord C, et al. Amygdala enlargement in toddlers with autism related to severity of social and communication impairments. Biol Psychiatry 2009;66(10):942–9.

64. Mosconi MW, Cody-Hazlett H, Poe MD, et al. Longitudinal study of amygdala volume and joint attention in 2- to 4-year-old children with autism. Arch Gen Psychiatry 2009;66(5):509–16.

65. Hazlett HC, Poe MD, Lightbody AA, et al. Teasing apart the heterogeneity of autism: same behavior, different brains in toddlers with fragile X syndrome and autism. J Neurodev Disord 2009;1(1):81–90.

66. Qiu T, Chang C, Li Y, et al. Two years changes in the development of caudate nucleus are involved in restricted repetitive behaviors in 2–5-year-old children with autism spectrum disorder. Dev Cogn Neurosci 2016;19:137–43.

67. Pote I, Wang S, Sethna V, et al. Familial risk of autism alters subcortical and cerebellar brain anatomy in infants and predicts the emergence of repetitive behaviors in early childhood. Autism Res 2019;12(4):614–27.

68. Fatemi SH, Aldinger KA, Ashwood P, et al. Consensus paper: pathological role of the cerebellum in autism. Cerebellum 2012;11(3):777–807.

69. Scott JA, Schumann CM, Goodlin-Jones BL, et al. A comprehensive volumetric analysis of the cerebellum in children and adolescents with autism spectrum disorder. Autism Res 2009; 2(5):246–57.

70. Webb SJ, Sparks B-F, Friedman SD, et al. Cerebellar vermal volumes and behavioral correlates in children with autism spectrum disorder. Psychiatry Res 2009;172(1):61–7.

71. Piven J, Saliba K, Bailey J, et al. An MRI study of autism: the cerebellum revisited. Neurology 1997; 49(2):546–51.

72. Manes F, Piven J, Vrancic D, et al. An MRI study of the corpus callosum and cerebellum in mentally retarded autistic individuals. J Neuropsychiatry Clin Neurosci 1999;11(4):470–4.

73. Frazier TW, Keshavan MS, Minshew NJ, et al. A two-year longitudinal MRI study of the corpus callosum in autism. J Autism Dev Disord 2012; 42(11):2312–22.

74. Boger-Megiddo I, Shaw DWW, Friedman SD, et al. Corpus callosum morphometrics in young children with autism spectrum disorder. J Autism Dev Disord 2006;36(6):733–9.

75. Nordahl CW, Iosif A-M, Young GS, et al. Sex differences in the corpus callosum in preschool-aged children with autism spectrum disorder. Mol Autism 2015;6(1):225.

76. Wolff JJ, Gerig G, Lewis JD, et al. Altered corpus callosum morphology associated with autism over the first 2 years of life. Brain 2015;138(Pt 7):2046–58.

77. Shen MD, Kim SH, McKinstry RC, et al. Increased extra-axial cerebrospinal fluid in high-risk infants who later develop autism. Biol Psychiatry 2017;82(3):186–93.

78. Shen MD, Nordahl CW, Li DD, et al. Extra-axial cerebrospinal fluid in high-risk and normal-risk children with autism aged 2–4 years: a case-control study. Lancet Psychiatry 2018. https://doi.org/10.1016/S2215-0366(18)30294-3.

79. Ben Bashat D, Kronfeld-Duenias V, Zachor DA, et al. Accelerated maturation of white matter in young children with autism: a high b value DWI study. Neuroimage 2007;37(1):40–7.

80. Dubois J, Dehaene-Lambertz G, Kulikova S, et al. The early development of brain white matter: a review of imaging studies in fetuses, newborns and infants. Neuroscience 2014;276:48–71.

81. Travers BG, Adluru N, Ennis C, et al. Diffusion tensor imaging in autism spectrum disorder: a review. Autism Res 2012;5(5):289–313.

82. Weinstein M, Ben Sira L, Levy Y, et al. Abnormal white matter integrity in young children with autism. Hum Brain Mapp 2011;32(4):534–43.

83. Conti E, Mitra J, Calderoni S, et al. Network overconnectivity differentiates autism spectrum disorder from other developmental disorders in toddlers: a diffusion MRI study. Hum Brain Mapp 2017;38(5):2333–44.

84. Jbabdi S, Johansen-Berg H. Tractography: where do we go from here? Brain Connect 2011;1(3):169–83.

85. Jones DK, Knösche TR, Turner R. White matter integrity, fiber count, and other fallacies: the do's and don'ts of diffusion MRI. Neuroimage 2013;73:239–54.

86. Fingher N, Dinstein I, Ben-Shachar M, et al. Toddlers later diagnosed with autism exhibit multiple structural abnormalities in temporal corpus callosum fibers. Cortex 2017;97:291–305.

87. Cascio C, Gribbin M, Gouttard S, et al. Fractional anisotropy distributions in 2- to 6-year-old children with autism. J Intellect Disabil Res 2013;57(11):1037–49.

88. Billeci L, Calderoni S, Tosetti M, et al. White matter connectivity in children with autism spectrum disorders: a tract-based spatial statistics study. BMC Neurol 2012;12(1):9228.

89. Wolff JJ, Gu H, Gerig G, et al. Differences in white matter fiber tract development present from 6 to 24 months in infants with autism. Am J Psychiatry 2012;169(6):589–600.

90. Solso S, Xu R, Proudfoot J, et al. Diffusion tensor imaging provides evidence of possible axonal overconnectivity in frontal lobes in autism spectrum disorder toddlers. Biol Psychiatry 2016;79(8):676–84.

91. Cao M, Huang H, He Y. Developmental connectomics from infancy through early childhood. Trends Neurosci 2017;40(8):494–506.

92. Lewis JD, Evans AC, Pruett JR, et al. Network inefficiencies in autism spectrum disorder at 24 months. Transl Psychiatry 2014;4(5):e388.

93. Lewis JD, Evans AC, Pruett JR, et al. The emergence of network inefficiencies in infants with autism spectrum disorder. Biol Psychiatry 2017;82(3):176–85.

94. Wolff JJ, Swanson MR, Elison JT, et al. Neural circuitry at age 6 months associated with later repetitive behavior and sensory responsiveness in autism. Mol Autism 2017;8(1):8.

95. Naigles LR, Johnson R, Mastergeorge A, et al. Neural correlates of language variability in preschool-aged boys with autism spectrum disorder. Autism Res 2017;44:2221.

96. Liu J, Tsang T, Jackson L, et al. Altered lateralization of dorsal language tracts in 6-week-old infants at risk for autism. Dev Sci 2019;22(3):e12768.

97. Redcay E, Courchesne E. Deviant functional magnetic resonance imaging patterns of brain activity to speech in 2-3-year-old children with autism spectrum disorder. Biol Psychiatry 2008;64(7):589–98.

98. Eyler LT, Pierce K, Courchesne E. A failure of left temporal cortex to specialize for language is an early emerging and fundamental property of autism. Brain 2012;135(3):949–60.

99. Dinstein I, Pierce K, Eyler L, et al. Disrupted neural synchronization in toddlers with autism. Neuron 2011;70(6):1218–25.

100. Lombardo MV, Pierce K, Eyler LT, et al. Different functional neural substrates for good and poor language outcome in autism. Neuron 2015;86(2):567–77.

101. Chen H, Wang J, Uddin LQ, et al. Aberrant functional connectivity of neural circuits associated with social and sensorimotor deficits in young children with autism spectrum disorder. Autism Res 2018;11(12):1643–52.

102. Ciarrusta J, O'Muircheartaigh J, Dimitrova R, et al. Social brain functional maturation in newborn infants with and without a family history of autism spectrum disorder. JAMA Netw Open 2019;2(4):e191868.

103. Shen MD, Li DD, Keown CL, et al. Functional connectivity of the amygdala is disrupted in

preschool-aged children with autism spectrum disorder. J Am Acad Child Adolesc Psychiatry 2016;55(9):817–24.

104. McKinnon CJ, Eggebrecht AT, Todorov A, et al. Restricted and repetitive behavior and brain functional connectivity in infants at risk for developing autism spectrum disorder. Biol Psychiatry Cogn Neurosci Neuroimaging 2019; 4(1):50–61.

105. Ozonoff S, Young GS, Belding A, et al. The broader autism phenotype in infancy: when does it emerge? J Am Acad Child Adolesc Psychiatry 2014;53(4):398–407.e2.

106. Knickmeyer RC, Gouttard S, Kang C, et al. A structural MRI study of human brain development from birth to 2 years. J Neurosci 2008; 28(47):12176–82.

107. Lui JH, Hansen DV, Kriegstein AR. Development and evolution of the human neocortex. Cell 2011; 146(1):18–36.

108. Nowakowski TJ, Pollen AA, Sandoval-Espinosa C, et al. Transformation of the radial glia scaffold demarcates two stages of human cerebral cortex development. Neuron 2016;91(6):1219–27.

109. Kriegstein A, Noctor S, Martínez-Cerdeño V. Patterns of neural stem and progenitor cell division may underlie evolutionary cortical expansion. Nat Rev Neurosci 2006;7(11):883–90.

110. Rakic P. A small step for the cell, a giant leap for mankind: a hypothesis of neocortical expansion during evolution. Trends Neurosci 1995;18(9): 383–8.

111. Silbereis JC, Pochareddy S, Zhu Y, et al. The cellular and molecular landscapes of the developing human central nervous system. Neuron 2016;89(2):248–68.

112. Packer A. Neocortical neurogenesis and the etiology of autism spectrum disorder. Neurosci Biobehav Rev 2016;64:185–95.

113. Marchetto MC, Belinson H, Tian Y, et al. Altered proliferation and networks in neural cells derived from idiopathic autistic individuals. Mol Psychiatry 2017;22(6):820–35.

114. Mariani J, Coppola G, Zhang P, et al. FOXG1-dependent dysregulation of GABA/glutamate neuron differentiation in autism spectrum disorders. Cell 2015;162(2):375–90.

115. Schafer ST, Paquola ACM, Stern S, et al. Pathological priming causes developmental gene network heterochronicity in autistic subject-derived neurons. Nat Neurosci 2019;22:345.

116. Kwon C-H, Luikart BW, Powell CM, et al. Pten regulates neuronal arborization and social interaction in mice. Neuron 2006;50(3):377–88.

117. Bernier R, Golzio C, Xiong B, et al. Disruptive CHD8 mutations define a subtype of autism early in development. Cell 2014;158(2):263–76.

118. Deshpande A, Yadav S, Dao DQ, et al. Cellular phenotypes in human iPSC-derived neurons from a genetic model of autism spectrum disorder. Cell Rep 2017;21(10):2678–87.

119. Qureshi AY, Mueller S, Snyder AZ, et al. Opposing brain differences in 16p11.2 deletion and duplication carriers. J Neurosci 2014;34(34):11199–211.

120. Fang W-Q, Chen W-W, Jiang L, et al. Overproduction of upper-layer neurons in the neocortex leads to autism-like features in mice. Cell Rep 2014; 9(5):1635–43.

121. Suetterlin P, Hurley S, Mohan C, et al. Altered neocortical gene expression, brain overgrowth and functional over-connectivity in chd8 haploinsufficient mice. Cereb Cortex 2018;28(6): 2192–206.

122. Piochon C, Kano M, Hansel C. LTD-like molecular pathways in developmental synaptic pruning. Nat Neurosci 2016;19(10):1299–310.

123. Hensch TK. Critical period plasticity in local cortical circuits. Nat Rev Neurosci 2005;6(11):877–88.

124. Huber KM, Gallagher SM, Warren ST, et al. Altered synaptic plasticity in a mouse model of fragile X mental retardation. Proc Natl Acad Sci U S A 2002;99(11):7746–50.

125. Auerbach BD, Osterweil EK, Bear MF. Mutations causing syndromic autism define an axis of synaptic pathophysiology. Nature 2011;480(7375): 63–8.

126. Baudouin SJ, Gaudias J, Gerharz S, et al. Shared synaptic pathophysiology in syndromic and non-syndromic rodent models of autism. Science 2012;338(6103):128–32.

127. Piochon C, Kloth AD, Grasselli G, et al. Cerebellar plasticity and motor learning deficits in a copy-number variation mouse model of autism. Nat Commun 2014;5(1):5586.

128. Shen MD. Cerebrospinal fluid and the early brain development of autism. J Neurodev Disord 2018; 10(1):893.

129. Lehtinen MK, Zappaterra MW, Chen X, et al. The cerebrospinal fluid provides a proliferative niche for neural progenitor cells. Neuron 2011;69(5): 893–905.

130. Johanson CE, Duncan JA, Klinge PM, et al. Multiplicity of cerebrospinal fluid functions: new challenges in health and disease. Cerebrospinal Fluid Res 2008;5(1):10.

131. Iliff JJ, Wang M, Liao Y, et al. A paravascular pathway facilitates CSF flow through the brain parenchyma and the clearance of interstitial solutes, including amyloid β. Sci Transl Med 2012;4(147): 147ra111.

132. Phan BN, Page SC, Campbell MN, et al. Defects of myelination are common pathophysiology in syndromic and idiopathic autism spectrum disorder. Biorxiv 2017;128124.

133. Lee H, Thacker S, Sarn N, et al. Constitutional mislocalization of Pten drives precocious maturation in oligodendrocytes and aberrant myelination in model of autism spectrum disorder. Transl Psychiatry 2019;9(1):13.

134. Zikopoulos B, Barbas H. Changes in prefrontal axons may disrupt the network in autism. J Neurosci 2010;30(44):14595–609.

135. Fields RD. A new mechanism of nervous system plasticity: activity-dependent myelination. Nat Rev Neurosci 2015;16(12):756–67.

136. Wake H, Ortiz FC, Woo DH, et al. Nonsynaptic junctions on myelinating glia promote preferential myelination of electrically active axons. Nat Commun 2015;6:7844.

137. Grove J, Ripke S, Als TD, et al. Identification of common genetic risk variants for autism spectrum disorder. Nat Genet 2019;51(3):431–44.

138. Courchesne E, Pramparo T, Gazestani VH, et al. The ASD Living Biology: from cell proliferation to clinical phenotype. Mol Psychiatry 2018;2(Pt 9):217.

139. Ozonoff S, Young GS, Steinfeld MB, et al. How early do parent concerns predict later autism diagnosis? J Dev Behav Pediatr 2009;30(5):367–75.

140. Chawarska K, Shic F, Macari S, et al. 18-month predictors of later outcomes in younger siblings of children with autism spectrum disorder: a baby siblings research consortium study. J Am Acad Child Adolesc Psychiatry 2014;53(12):1317–27.e1.

141. Pandey J, Verbalis A, Robins DL, et al. Screening for autism in older and younger toddlers with the modified checklist for autism in toddlers. Autism 2008;12(5):513–35.

142. Zwaigenbaum L, Bryson S, Lord C, et al. Clinical assessment and management of toddlers with suspected autism spectrum disorder: insights from studies of high-risk infants. Pediatrics 2009; 123(5):1383–91.

143. Vieira S, Pinaya WHL, Mechelli A. Using deep learning to investigate the neuroimaging correlates of psychiatric and neurological disorders: methods and applications. Neurosci Biobehav Rev 2017;74: 58–75.

144. Pereira F, Mitchell T, Botvinick M. Machine learning classifiers and fMRI: a tutorial overview. Neuroimage 2009;45(1 Suppl):S199–209.

145. Mostapha M, Styner M. Role of deep learning in infant brain MRI analysis. Magn Reson Imaging 2019. https://doi.org/10.1016/j.mri.2019.06.009.

146. Chawla NV, Bowyer KW, Hall LO, et al. SMOTE: synthetic minority over-sampling technique. J Artif Intell 2002;16:321–57.

147. Taft LM, Evans RS, Shyu CR, et al. Countering imbalanced datasets to improve adverse drug event predictive models in labor and delivery. J Biomed Inform 2009;42(2):356–64.

148. Shen MD, Piven J. Brain and behavior development in autism from birth through infancy. Dialogues Clin Neurosci 2017;19(4):325–33.

149. Gabrieli JDE, Ghosh SS, Whitfield-Gabrieli S. Prediction as a humanitarian and pragmatic contribution from human cognitive neuroscience. Neuron 2015;85(1):11–26.

150. Danhong W, Meiling L, Meiyun W, et al. Individual-specific functional connectivity markers track dimensional and categorical features of psychotic illness. Mol Psychiatry 2018. https://doi.org/10.1038/s41380-018-0276-1.

151. Huang X, Gong Q, Sweeney JA, et al. Progress in psychoradiology, the clinical application of psychiatric neuroimaging. Br J Radiol 2019;92(1101): 20181000.

152. Lei D, Pinaya WHL, van Amelsvoort T, et al. Detecting schizophrenia at the level of the individual: relative diagnostic value of whole-brain images, connectome-wide functional connectivity and graph-based metrics. Psychol Med 2019;1–10. https://doi.org/10.1017/S0033291719001934.

153. Port JD. Diagnosis of attention deficit hyperactivity disorder by using MR imaging and radiomics: a potential tool for clinicians. Radiology 2018;287: 631–2.

154. Sun H, Chen Y, Huang Q, et al. Psychoradiologic utility of MR imaging for diagnosis of attention deficit hyperactivity disorder: a radiomics analysis. Radiology 2018;287(2):620–30.

155. Collins FS, Varmus H. A new initiative on precision medicine. N Engl J Med 2015;372(9):793–5.

156. Estes A, Munson J, Rogers SJ, et al. Long-term outcomes of early intervention in 6-year-old children with autism spectrum disorder. J Am Acad Child Adolesc Psychiatry 2015;54(7): 580–7.

157. Dawson G, Rogers S, Munson J, et al. Randomized, controlled trial of an intervention for toddlers with autism: the early start Denver model. Pediatrics 2010;125(1):e17–23.

158. Kasari C, Gulsrud A, Paparella T, et al. Randomized comparative efficacy study of parent-mediated interventions for toddlers with autism. J Consult Clin Psychol 2015;83(3):554–63.

159. Howlin P, Magiati I, Charman T. Systematic review of early intensive behavioral interventions for children with autism. Am J Intellect Dev Disabil 2009; 114(1):23–41.

160. Whitehouse AJO, Varcin KJ, Alvares GA, et al. Pre-emptive intervention versus treatment as usual for infants showing early behavioural risk signs of autism spectrum disorder: a single-blind, randomised controlled trial. Lancet Child Adolesc Health 2019;3(9):605–15.

161. Girault JB, Munsell BC, Puechmaille D, et al. White matter connectomes at birth accurately predict

cognitive abilities at age 2. Neuroimage 2019;192: 145–55.

162. Kawahara J, Brown CJ, Miller SP, et al. Brain-NetCNN: convolutional neural networks for brain networks; towards predicting neurodevelopment. Neuroimage 2017;146:1038–49.

163. Constantino JN. Early behavioral indices of inherited liability to autism. Pediatr Res 2018;114(5 Pt 2):129.

164. Constantino JN, Charman T. Diagnosis of autism spectrum disorder: reconciling the syndrome, its diverse origins, and variation in expression. Lancet Neurol 2016;15(3):279–91.

165. Feczko E, Balba NM, Miranda-Dominguez O, et al. Subtyping cognitive profiles in autism spectrum disorder using a functional random forest algorithm. Neuroimage 2018;172:674–88.

166. Gates KM, Molenaar PCM, Iyer SP, et al. Organizing heterogeneous samples using community detection of GIMME-derived resting state functional networks. PLoS One 2014;9(3):e91322.

167. Gordon EM, Laumann TO, Adeyemo B, et al. Individual-specific features of brain systems identified with resting state functional correlations. Neuroimage 2017;146:918–39.

168. Gates KM, Molenaar PCM. Group search algorithm recovers effective connectivity maps for individuals in homogeneous and heterogeneous samples. Neuroimage 2012;63(1):310–9.

169. Insel TR. The NIMH research domain criteria (RDoC) project: precision medicine for psychiatry. Am J Psychiatry 2014;171(4):395–7.

170. Jacob S, Wolff JJ, Steinbach MS, et al. Neurodevelopmental heterogeneity and computational approaches for understanding autism. Transl Psychiatry 2019;9(1):63.

171. Gaugler T, Klei L, Sanders SJ, et al. Most genetic risk for autism resides with common variation. Nat Genet 2014;46(8):881–5.

172. Boyle EA, Li YI, Pritchard JK. An expanded view of complex traits: from polygenic to omnigenic. Cell 2017;169(7):1177–86.

173. Weiner DJ, Wigdor EM, Ripke S, et al. Polygenic transmission disequilibrium confirms that common and rare variation act additively to create risk for autism spectrum disorders. Nat Genet 2017; 49(7):978–85.

174. Moreno-De-Luca A, Evans DW, Boomer KB, et al. The role of parental cognitive, behavioral, and motor profiles in clinical variability in individuals with chromosome 16p11.2 deletions. JAMA Psychiatry 2015;72(2):119–26.

175. LeBarton ES, Landa RJ. Infant motor skill predicts later expressive language and autism spectrum disorder diagnosis. Infant Behav Dev 2019;54: 37–47.

176. Bhat AN, Galloway JC, Landa RJ. Relation between early motor delay and later communication delay in infants at risk for autism. Infant Behav Dev 2012;35(4):838–46.

177. Bedford R, Pickles A, Lord C. Early gross motor skills predict the subsequent development of language in children with autism spectrum disorder. Autism Res 2016;9(9):993–1001.

178. Gopalakrishnan J. The emergence of stem cell-based brain organoids: trends and challenges. Bioessays 2019;41(8):e1900011.

Imaging of Posttraumatic Stress Disorder

Kouhei Kamiya, MD, PhD*, Osamu Abe, MD, PhD

KEYWORDS

- Diffusion MR imaging • Functional MR imaging • Psychoradiology • Posttraumatic stress disorder
- Structural MR imaging

KEY POINTS

- The most robustly identified findings in posttraumatic stress disorder (PTSD) include hyperactivation of the amygdala and dorsal anterior cingulate cortex, hypoactivation of the ventromedial prefrontal cortex, and atrophy of the hippocampus.
- Functional disruption of these brain regions is thought to impair neurocircuits for fear learning, threat detection, contextual processing, executive function, and emotional regulation in PTSD.
- In the triple-network model, PTSD is characterized by hypoactivation of the default mode network (DMN) and central executive network (CEN) and overactivation of the salience network (SN).
- Hyperactivation of the SN is thought to result in hypersensitive threat detection, as well as inefficient modulation of the DMN and CEN.

INTRODUCTION

Posttraumatic stress disorder (PTSD) is a common neuropsychological disorder that presents a large burden to society in terms of both treatment cost and loss of productivity.[1] People with PTSD suffer from persistent symptoms, vivid re-experiencing of traumatic events, avoidance, negative thoughts and feelings, and hyperarousal.[2] PTSD can result from various kinds of severely stressful events, including military combat and natural disasters. PTSD differs from other psychological disorders in that the causes are readily identified. Its prevalence varies substantially with social background; for example, the prevalence is estimated to be 6.8% in the general population in the United States[3] but 23% in US veterans.[4] Since the establishment of PTSD as a formal diagnostic entity in the American psychiatric nomenclature in 1980,[5] the number of published neuroimaging studies in PTSD has grown rapidly. The traditional fronto-limbic model of PTSD first proposed by Rauch and colleagues[6] in 1998 suggested that the underlying dysfunctions in PTSD are hypoactivation of the medial prefrontal cortex (mPFC), resulting in loss of inhibitory control of the limbic system, and hyperactivity of the amygdala and abnormal functioning of the hippocampus.[7,8] Since the proposal of the fronto-limbic model, several neurocircuits that modulate the recognition and expression of fear and the response to threat have been implicated in PTSD.[9,10] Recent studies have also identified the involvement of regions outside the fronto-limbic system and the impairment of broader networks.[11–14] The traditional model focusing on fear, although a powerful and useful framework, is thought to be insufficient to explain the full range of symptoms patients experience (e.g., emotional numbing, avoidance, dissociation) and neuroimaging findings.[2,15] In the past 2 decades, our understanding of PTSD has evolved greatly and rapidly through the integration of preclinical and clinical research,[10,16,17] and neuroimaging has played a key role in this process by identifying several neuronal circuits and their relevance to the pathogenesis.

Disclosure Statement: This research was supported by "Brain/MINDS and Beyond" Grant Number: JP18dm0307001. The authors have no financial disclosure related to this work.
Department of Radiology, University of Tokyo, 7-3-1 Hongo, Bunkyo-ku, Tokyo 113-8655, Japan
* Corresponding author.
E-mail address: kkamiya-tky@umin.ac.jp

neuroimaging.theclinics.com

This review summarizes the knowledge from psychoradiological studies of PTSD. We first describe key anatomic structures that have been robustly implicated in PTSD. Then, we introduce widely accepted concepts supporting neurobiological models of PTSD. These concepts explain the vast majority of reported neuroimaging findings, their interactions, and their relationships to the functional disruptions in PTSD. In the last part of this review, we discuss the limitations of current psychoradiological studies that need to be addressed in future research.

LOCAL NEUROIMAGING FINDINGS IDENTIFIED IN POSTTRAUMATIC STRESS DISORDER

Key anatomic structures have been consistently implicated in PTSD since the early days of neuroimaging research into the disorder. These include 3 brain regions that are involved in memory functioning and stress response: the hippocampus, amygdala, and mPFC[6–8] (**Fig. 1**).

Hippocampus

Memory disturbances, that is, intrusive memories and deficits in declarative memory function, are characteristic features of PTSD.[8] The hippocampus plays a central role in declarative memory, and thus its impairment has been postulated in PTSD. The hippocampus is also known to play a crucial role in the biological response to stress.[18] Indeed, since the pioneering studies,[19,20] the most replicated structural MR imaging finding in PTSD is a smaller hippocampal volume compared with controls.[21–26] Volumetric studies further focusing on the subfields of the hippocampus found that PTSD, in both adults[27] and adolescents,[28] is associated with

selective volume loss of cornu ammonis (CA) 2 to 3 and the dentate gyrus that is negatively correlated with intrusion symptoms. Studies using magnetic resonance spectroscopy have consistently found smaller amounts of N-acetylaspartate in the hippocampi of the patients, possibly indicating reduced neuronal density.[29] Meta-analyses of functional MR imaging (fMR imaging) studies[12,13] yielded mixed results, with studies reporting either higher or lower hippocampus activity in patients than in controls.

Amygdala

The amygdala is a key structure for the recognition of danger, response to fear, emotion, and motivation.[8,30] Fear-related memory formation has been localized to the amygdala; subsequent modulations, such as extinction or safety learning, have been further localized to the basolateral complex (BLC) of the amygdala.[10] In addition, the BLC provides the main input to the central nucleus, the source of the outputs that lead to physiologic and behavioral expressions of fear.[10] In PTSD, fMR imaging studies have robustly found higher amygdala activity in patients than in controls.[12–14] Results from MR imaging volumetry studies are mixed, with studies reporting larger, smaller, or unchanged volumes of the amygdala in patients with PTSD.[23,26,31–33]

Medial Prefrontal Cortex

Within the mPFC, 2 subregions have been robustly implicated in PTSD: the dorsal anterior cingulate cortex (dACC) and the ventromedial prefrontal cortex (vmPFC), homologues of the prelimbic cortex and infralimbic cortex in rodents. In general, the volume of the mPFC is smaller in patients with PTSD.[23,24] As we will see later, dACC and vmPFC show distinct functional abnormalities in PTSD,

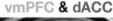
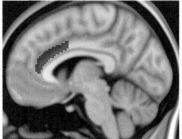

Amygdala	**Hippocampus**	**vmPFC & dACC**
• Activation ↑ • Volume ↑↓	• Volume ↓ • NAA ↓ • Activation ↑↓	• Volume ↓ • vmPFC activation ↓ • dACC activation ↑

Fig. 1. The most robustly identified neuroimaging abnormalities in PTSD. An upward and downward arrow indicates greater and smaller values, respectively, as compared to the normal controls. The presence of both two arrows mean the previous studies reported inconsistent results for that metric. NAA, N-acetylaspartate.

which can be understood in the contexts of circuits/networks relevant to the symptoms.

NEUROBIOLOGICAL MODELS OF POSTTRAUMATIC STRESS DISORDER

Psychiatric disorders in general are becoming understood as involving multiscale, multidimensional neural networks rather than isolated impairment of local brain regions.[34,35] Here we introduce widely accepted concepts about the neurobiological circuits and networks involved in PTSD. Because these concepts are based on the same body of literature, they are not mutually exclusive but rather are overlapping and complementary.

The Brain Functional Circuits Impaired in Posttraumatic Stress Disorder

The neuronal circuits impaired in PTSD include those responsible for fear learning, threat detection, contextual processing, executive function, and emotional regulation.[9,10,12] The neuroimaging findings about these circuits in humans are strikingly similar to observations in the homologous brain structures in rodents,[10,16] representing a successful example of translational neuroscience. More comprehensive reviews on these neurocircuits, including evidence from animal studies, can be found in Refs.[9,10,16]

Fear learning
The persistence of fear responses in patients with PTSD has been attributed not only to fear-related memory but also to impaired extinction (learning safety) and extinction recall.[36] Appropriate extinction and fear expression requires a network among nuclei within the amygdala,[10,37] as well as coordination with other brain regions. Studies in healthy humans have implicated the vmPFC and hippocampus in extinction[38] and the dACC in fear expression.[39] Functional neuroimaging studies in PTSD[12–14,36,40–44] found that the dACC and amygdala were hyperactivated in patients, whereas the vmPFC and the hippocampus were hypoactivated. In addition, decreased vmPFC activity in the patients was associated with increased amygdala activity.[13,36]

Threat detection
Hypersensitive threat detection is considered to underlie the heightened vigilance, threat reactivity, and protective responses that are disproportionate to actual threats in PTSD.[45] Functional neuroimaging studies have identified brain regions that respond to threats and salience in general, including the amygdala, the dACC, and the insula.[46,47] PTSD has been associated with hyperactivity of these brain regions,[12–14,39] which is consistent with its symptoms. In addition, a smaller anterior cingulate cortex (ACC) volume has been robustly reported in PTSD and may underpin the attentional deficits and inability to modulate emotions.[26]

Contextual processing
The hypervigilance inappropriate to the situation and difficulty in differentiating safety from threat[48] in PTSD is considered to result from improper contextual processing.[10] The vmPFC, the hippocampus, and the thalamus are important for appropriate contextual processing.[49,50] As we described previously, smaller hippocampal and vmPFC volumes have been implicated in PTSD.[19–26] Diminished functional activity of the vmPFC in patients with PTSD has been linked to abnormal processing of contextual information,[40] as well as to impaired extinction recall[36] as discussed previously.

Executive function and emotion regulation
Impaired executive function and emotion regulation have been suspected to underlie memory and concentration deficits, poor control of emotional responses, irritability, and impulsivity in PTSD.[9,10] Meta-analyses of fMR imaging studies[12–14] confirmed diminished activity in the dorsolateral PFC (dlPFC), which is crucial for cognitive control of thought, emotion, working memory, and behavior.[51,52] Interestingly, whereas decreased cortical thickness has been reported in cross-sectional studies of patients,[53,54] a longitudinal study[55] reported increased dlPFC thickness approximately 1 year after trauma, possibly reflecting the increased burden of emotional regulation.

Triple-Network Model

Neuroimaging studies in PTSD have typically identified impairments in several regions outside the circuits referred to previously, such as the posterior cingulate cortex (PCC).[44,45] Recently, increasing evidence from neuroimaging studies (for reviews see Refs.[11,13,14]) supported that the functional impairments in PTSD can be explained from the perspective of the triple-network model of Menon.[52] This theory proposes that a wide range of psychological disorders can be understood as a disruption of 3 core neurocognitive networks: the default mode network (DMN), the central executive network (CEN), and the salience network (SN) (Fig. 2), which is in accordance with the psychoradiological hypothesis by Gong and colleagues, theorizing that brain structural alteration leads to clinical syndromes via impact on widely distributed functional connectivity.[34,57–59]

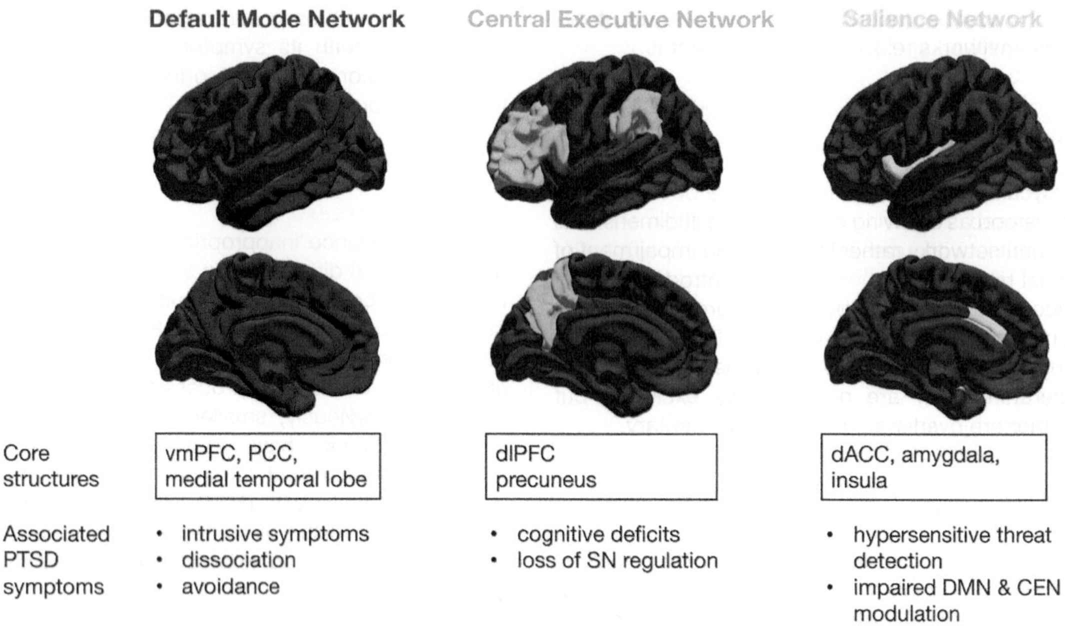

Fig. 2. The triple-network model of PTSD. The figure shows the core anatomic structures of the DMN, CEN, and SN, as well as the characteristic symptoms of PTSD that are putatively linked to disruption of each network. The illustrations on the brain surface were generated using FreeSurfer software and the Desikan-Killiany Atlas.[56]

Default mode network

The core regions of the DMN are the vmPFC, PCC, and the medial temporal lobes, including the hippocampus. Other structures such as the lateral temporal lobe and the posterior inferior parietal lobule are also involved. The DMN is suppressed during externally oriented, attention-demanding tasks relative to its activity in the resting state.[60] The main functions of the DMN are thought to involve self-referential thoughts and other introspective processes, which are activities that predominantly occur at rest. A malfunction of the DMN has therefore been postulated to explain the intrusive symptoms, dissociation, and avoidance seen in patients with PTSD[2]; this proposed malfunction has been supported by studies that link altered self-referential processing in patients with PTSD with dysregulation of DMN.[61,62] Resting-state fMR imaging connectivity studies in PTSD have demonstrated decreased coupling between structures of the DMN, such as between the vmPFC and hippocampus,[45] PCC and hippocampus,[62] and PCC and vmPFC.[62] Diffusion MR imaging studies have found lower fractional anisotropy values in the white matter of the vmPFC region[63] and in the white matter linking the vmPFC to the PCC (cingulum)[64–66] and to the hippocampus.[66,67]

Central executive network

The CEN comprises the dlPFC, anterior inferior parietal lobule, precuneus, and part of the premotor cortex. It underpins goal-directed behavior, working memory, and emotional control.[47] Disruption of the CEN is postulated to result in the cognitive deficits and loss of top-down emotional control observed in PTSD.[52] fMR imaging connectivity studies[61,68] have linked aberrant functional connectivity within the CEN with cognitive dysfunction in PTSD.

Salience network

The SN is anchored in the insula and dACC, with extensive connectivity to subcortical regions including the amygdala, thalamus, ventral striatopallidum, and substantia nigra/ventral tegmental area.[47] The SN is associated with detection of stimuli, as well as with homoeostatic regulation, interoception, autonomic function, and reward processing. In addition, the SN is thought to modulate the dynamics of the DMN and CEN (switching between task-relevant and task-irrelevant behavior), mediated predominantly by the anterior insular cortex.[69,70] The anterior insula and dACC are hyperactive in patients with PTSD,[12,13,39] suggesting that overactivity of the SN is responsible for the heightened threat detection and autonomic dysfunction. The hyperactivity of the anterior part of insula possibly leads to loss of appropriate control of the limbic system by the prefrontal region or to impaired modulation of the DMN and CEN.[61,68] In contrast to the anterior insula, the posterior insula is hypoactive.[12,14]

The neurobiological evidence from the interactions within and among these functional networks also supports a dissociative subtype of PTSD.[71,72] Studies of neurobiological responses to traumatic symptom provocation have indicated that, although the "classic" PTSD is associated with decreased activity of vmPFC and increased activity of the amygdala and insula, patients with dissociative PTSD exhibit the opposite pattern: increased vmPFC activity and decreased amygdala and insula activity.[72,73] These subtypes are considered to be different extremes of emotional dysregulation caused by underinhibition and overinhibition of the limbic system by vmPFC. In line with this, a recent resting-state fMR imaging study reported that patients with dissociative PTSD exhibited greater functional connectivity from the amygdala to the prefrontal regions involved in emotional regulation and to the parietal regions involved in consciousness, awareness, and proprioception, compared with individuals with "classic" PTSD.[74] Further investigation of these PTSD subtypes is of clinical importance, because the best treatment strategy may vary between the subtypes.[17]

Some of the reported findings are yet not completely explained by this triple network, and further expansion and modification may be needed. For example, abnormal activation in sensory cortex[12] and other sensory pathologies[75] have been implicated in PTSD, and a recent fMR imaging study[76] postulated a vicious cycle in which the circuit among the sensory cortex, prefrontal cortex, and amygdala is dysregulated, such that hyperactivity in the sensory cortex overloads the frontal cortex, disrupting executive control.

LIMITATIONS AND FUTURE DIRECTIONS

Despite the rapid progress in neuroimaging techniques and the disease model of PTSD, imaging has not yet provided a reliable, clinically useful biomarker or led to a large change in therapeutic strategies.[17,77] In the following sections we describe 2 major limitations hampering complete elucidation of the pathogenesis and direct translation to clinical practice. As we have seen, considerable work has already been done using the widely available MR imaging sequences and cross-sectional case-control study designs, and there may be little more to gain from these approaches. The following limitations are not merely a matter of effect size and statistical power but rather are fundamental to neuroimaging of psychological disorders. We therefore need to rethink

the boundaries of diagnostic clusters in view of the biological evidence,[78,79] as well as to promote communication with other fields, including genetics, molecular neuroscience, network science, engineering, computer science, and statistics.[17,79]

Diagnostic Criteria and Heterogeneity Within the Disease

Human neuroimaging studies almost always rely on clinical diagnostic criteria as a "gold standard." However, because PTSD was established as a diagnosis more recently than other psychological disorders, the diagnostic criteria for PTSD have been subject to dramatic revisions in recent years. In the fifth edition of the American Psychiatric Association's *Diagnostic and Statistical Manual of Mental Disorders* (DSM-5),[2] avoidance has been added as one of the required diagnostic clusters, and negative cognitions are highlighted. Such modifications in diagnostic criteria have great influence on both clinical practice and research.[80] One study reported that the overlap between persons identified as having PTSD according to the DSM-IV[81] and DSM-5[2] was only 55%.[82] It is unclear to what extent we can apply the findings of previous studies that used older diagnostic criteria to the population diagnosed with newer criteria. Also, inclusion of the dissociative subtype of PTSD in DSM-5 confirms the considerable heterogeneity included under the same diagnosis. In addition, the real patient population in the clinics is far more complex than the "clean" study population used in research, with a high prevalence of comorbidities like depression and heterogeneities in social background and medications.

Predisposing Risk Factors or Products of the Disorder?

Do the neuroimaging findings in PTSD represent genetic or environmental risk factors causing vulnerability to the disease, or secondary alterations resulting from the traumatic event and/or the chronic disability? The distinction between preexisting and acquired abnormalities is crucial for disease monitoring and discovery of novel therapies, but our knowledge is currently limited on this front. It is now widely accepted that various genetic factors contribute to PTSD risk.[83] Structural MR imaging studies of monozygotic twins have suggested that the smaller hippocampal volume in PTSD is a pretrauma risk factor.[84] However, stress also causes loss of hippocampal volume,[85,86] which can be reversible after a certain time without stress exposure.[87] Indeed, clinical improvement after cognitive behavioral therapy in

PTSD is reported to be associated with an increase in hippocampal volume.[88] The volume change in the hippocampus may be a mixture of both predisposing factors and dynamic changes after trauma. Similarly, we have not yet reached a clear distinction between causes and effects in the medial prefrontal region. Although a study of combat-discordant twins suggested that the smaller volume of the ventral ACC is an acquired deficit,[89] a study of subjects who underwent MR imaging before and after an earthquake found that the volume of the ventral ACC before the earthquake was negatively associated with PTSD symptoms.[90] Twin studies using fMR imaging suggested that increased amygdala and dACC activity in fear learning is a predisposing risk factor for PTSD, whereas diminished activation of mPFC during recollection of stressful events[91] and reduced functional connectivity between the mPFC and hippocampus[92,93] are acquired dysfunctions. To address this issue of causes and effects by using neuroimaging, a pretrauma, prospective, and longitudinal study is necessary, although such study would be expensive and difficult to perform.

SUMMARY

Neuroimaging has contributed greatly to our current understanding of PTSD. Today, most neuroimaging findings are interpreted in the context of brain networks, and evidence from clinical and preclinical studies is beginning to converge toward a unifying biological model of PTSD. It is now widely accepted that PTSD is characterized by hypoactivation of the DMN and CEN and overactivation of the SN. At the same time, we must acknowledge the discrepancy between such remarkable scientific progress and the limited application in clinical practice. To break down the barriers for clinical translation, our research model needs to be updated with active communication with other fields of science. In particular, the development of psychoradiology, an emerging subspecialty of radiology,[34,94–97] has shown promise in bringing psychiatric imaging into clinical care such as guiding diagnosis and treatment planning for psychiatric patients.

REFERENCES

1. Kessler RC. Posttraumatic stress disorder: the burden to the individual and to society. J Clin Psychiatry 2000;61(Suppl 5):4–12 [discussion: 13–4]. Available at: http://www.ncbi.nlm.nih.gov/pubmed/10761674.

2. American Psychiatric Association. Diagnostic and statistical manual of mental disorders (DSM-5®). Arlington (VA): American Psychiatric Pub; 2013.

3. Kessler RC, Berglund P, Demler O, et al. Lifetime prevalence and age-of-onset distributions of DSM-IV disorders in the National Comorbidity Survey Replication. Arch Gen Psychiatry 2005;62(6): 593–602.

4. Fulton JJ, Calhoun PS, Wagner HR, et al. The prevalence of posttraumatic stress disorder in Operation Enduring Freedom/Operation Iraqi Freedom (OEF/OIF) Veterans: a meta-analysis. J Anxiety Disord 2015;31:98–107.

5. American Psychiatric Association. Diagnostic and statistical manual of mental disorders (DSM-3). Washington, DC: APA Publishing; 1980.

6. Rauch SL, Shin LM, Whalen PJ, et al. Neuroimaging and the neuroanatomy of posttraumatic stress disorder. CNS Spectr 1998;3(S2):30–41.

7. Rauch SL, Shin LM, Phelps EA. Neurocircuitry models of posttraumatic stress disorder and extinction: human neuroimaging research–past, present, and future. Biol Psychiatry 2006;60(4):376–82.

8. Elzinga BM, Bremner JD. Are the neural substrates of memory the final common pathway in posttraumatic stress disorder (PTSD)? J Affect Disord 2002;70(1):1–17. Available at: http://www.ncbi.nlm.nih.gov/pubmed/12113915.

9. Shalev A, Liberzon I, Marmar C. Post-traumatic stress disorder. N Engl J Med 2017;376(25): 2459–69.

10. Liberzon I, Abelson JL. Context processing and the neurobiology of post-traumatic stress disorder. Neuron 2016;92(1):14–30.

11. Akiki TJ, Averill CL, Abdallah CG. A network-based neurobiological model of PTSD: evidence from structural and functional neuroimaging studies. Curr Psychiatry Rep 2017;19(11). https://doi.org/10.1007/s11920-017-0840-4.

12. Patel R, Spreng RN, Shin LM, et al. Neurocircuitry models of posttraumatic stress disorder and beyond: a meta-analysis of functional neuroimaging studies. Neurosci Biobehav Rev 2012;36(9): 2130–42.

13. Hayes JP, Hayes SM, Mikedis AM. Quantitative meta-analysis of neural activity in posttraumatic stress disorder. Biol Mood Anxiety Disord 2012;2:9.

14. Koch SBJ, van Zuiden M, Nawijn L, et al. Aberrant resting-state brain activity in posttraumatic stress disorder: a meta-analysis and systematic review. Depress Anxiety 2016;33(7):592–605.

15. Resick PA, Miller MW. Posttraumatic stress disorder: anxiety or traumatic stress disorder? J Trauma Stress 2009;22(5):384–90.

16. Milad MR, Quirk GJ. Fear extinction as a model for translational neuroscience: ten years of progress. Annu Rev Psychol 2012;63:129–51.

17. Fenster RJ, Lebois LAM, Ressler KJ, et al. Brain circuit dysfunction in post-traumatic stress disorder: from mouse to man. Nat Rev Neurosci 2018;19(9): 535–51.

18. Sapolsky RM. Glucocorticoids and hippocampal atrophy in neuropsychiatric disorders. Arch Gen Psychiatry 2000;57(10):925–35. Available at: http://www.ncbi.nlm.nih.gov/pubmed/11015810.

19. Bremner JD, Randall P, Scott TM, et al. MRI-based measurement of hippocampal volume in patients with combat-related posttraumatic stress disorder. Am J Psychiatry 1995;152(7):973–81.

20. Gurvits TV, Shenton ME, Hokama H, et al. Magnetic resonance imaging study of hippocampal volume in chronic, combat-related posttraumatic stress disorder. Biol Psychiatry 1996;40(11):1091–9.

21. Kitayama N, Vaccarino V, Kutner M, et al. Magnetic resonance imaging (MRI) measurement of hippocampal volume in posttraumatic stress disorder: a meta-analysis. J Affect Disord 2005;88(1):79–86.

22. Smith ME. Bilateral hippocampal volume reduction in adults with post-traumatic stress disorder: a meta-analysis of structural MRI studies. Hippocampus 2005;15(6):798–807.

23. Karl A, Schaefer M, Malta LS, et al. A meta-analysis of structural brain abnormalities in PTSD. Neurosci Biobehav Rev 2006;30(7):1004–31.

24. Bromis K, Calem M, Reinders AATS, et al. Meta-analysis of 89 structural MRI studies in posttraumatic stress disorder and comparison with major depressive disorder. Am J Psychiatry 2018; 175(10):989–98.

25. Logue MW, van Rooij SJH, Dennis EL, et al. Smaller hippocampal volume in posttraumatic stress disorder: a multisite ENIGMA-PGC study: subcortical volumetry results from Posttraumatic Stress Disorder Consortia. Biol Psychiatry 2018;83(3):244–53.

26. O'Doherty DCM, Chitty KM, Saddiqui S, et al. A systematic review and meta-analysis of magnetic resonance imaging measurement of structural volumes in posttraumatic stress disorder. Psychiatry Res Neuroimaging 2015;232(1):1–33.

27. Wang Z, Neylan TC, Mueller SG, et al. Magnetic resonance imaging of hippocampal subfields in posttraumatic stress disorder. Arch Gen Psychiatry 2010;67(3):296–303.

28. Postel C, Viard A, André C, et al. Hippocampal subfields alterations in adolescents with post-traumatic stress disorder. Hum Brain Mapp 2018;1–9. https://doi.org/10.1002/hbm.24443.

29. Quadrelli S, Mountford C, Ramadan S. Systematic review of in-vivo neuro magnetic resonance spectroscopy for the assessment of posttraumatic stress disorder. Psychiatry Res Neuroimaging 2018;282: 110–25.

30. Janak PH, Tye KM. From circuits to behaviour in the amygdala. Nature 2015;517(7534):284–92.

31. Kuo JR, Kaloupek DG, Woodward SH. Amygdala volume in combat-exposed veterans with and without posttraumatic stress disorder: a cross-sectional study. Arch Gen Psychiatry 2012;69(10): 1080–6.

32. Morey RA, Gold AL, LaBar KS, et al. Amygdala volume changes in posttraumatic stress disorder in a large case-controlled veterans group. Arch Gen Psychiatry 2012;69(11):1169–78.

33. Woon FL, Hedges DW. Amygdala volume in adults with posttraumatic stress disorder: a meta-analysis. J Neuropsychiatry Clin Neurosci 2009;21(1): 5–12.

34. Lui S, Zhou XJ, Sweeney JA, et al. Psychoradiology: the frontier of neuroimaging in psychiatry. Radiology 2016;281(2):357–72.

35. Braun U, Schaefer A, Betzel RF, et al. From maps to multi-dimensional network mechanisms of mental disorders. Neuron 2018;97(1):14–31.

36. Milad MR, Pitman RK, Ellis CB, et al. Neurobiological basis of failure to recall extinction memory in posttraumatic stress disorder. Biol Psychiatry 2009; 66(12):1075–82.

37. Phelps EA, Delgado MR, Nearing KI, et al. Extinction learning in humans: role of the amygdala and vmPFC. Neuron 2004;43(6):897–905.

38. Milad MR, Wright CI, Orr SP, et al. Recall of fear extinction in humans activates the ventromedial prefrontal cortex and hippocampus in concert. Biol Psychiatry 2007;62(5):446–54.

39. Milad MR, Quirk GJ, Pitman RK, et al. A role for the human dorsal anterior cingulate cortex in fear expression. Biol Psychiatry 2007;62(10):1191–4.

40. Rougemont-Bücking A, Linnman C, Zeffiro TA, et al. Altered processing of contextual information during fear extinction in PTSD: an fMRI study. CNS Neurosci Ther 2011;17(4):227–36.

41. Shin LM, Shin PS, Heckers S, et al. Hippocampal function in posttraumatic stress disorder. Hippocampus 2004;14(3):292–300.

42. Shin LM, Whalen PJ, Pitman RK, et al. An fMRI study of anterior cingulate function in posttraumatic stress disorder. Biol Psychiatry 2001;50(12): 932–42. Available at: http://www.ncbi.nlm.nih.gov/pubmed/11750889.

43. Bryant RA, Felmingham KL, Kemp AH, et al. Neural networks of information processing in posttraumatic stress disorder: a functional magnetic resonance imaging study. Biol Psychiatry 2005;58(2):111–8.

44. Lanius RA, Frewen PA, Girotti M, et al. Neural correlates of trauma script-imagery in posttraumatic stress disorder with and without comorbid major depression: a functional MRI investigation. Psychiatry Res 2007;155(1):45–56.

45. Sripada RK, King AP, Welsh RC, et al. Neural dysregulation in posttraumatic stress disorder: evidence for disrupted equilibrium between salience and

default mode brain networks. Psychosom Med 2012;74(9):904–11.

46. Paulus MP, Stein MB. An insular view of anxiety. Biol Psychiatry 2006;60(4):383–7.

47. Seeley WW, Menon V, Schatzberg AF, et al. Dissociable intrinsic connectivity networks for salience processing and executive control. J Neurosci 2007;27(9):2349–56.

48. Grillon C, Morgan CA, Davis M, et al. Effects of experimental context and explicit threat cues on acoustic startle in Vietnam veterans with posttraumatic stress disorder. Biol Psychiatry 1998; 44(10):1027–36. Available at: http://www.ncbi.nlm.nih.gov/pubmed/9821567.

49. Lang S, Kroll A, Lipinski SJ, et al. Context conditioning and extinction in humans: differential contribution of the hippocampus, amygdala and prefrontal cortex. Eur J Neurosci 2009;29(4):823–32.

50. Maren S, Phan KL, Liberzon I. The contextual brain: implications for fear conditioning, extinction and psychopathology. Nat Rev Neurosci 2013;14(6): 417–28.

51. Weber DL, Clark CR, McFarlane AC, et al. Abnormal frontal and parietal activity during working memory updating in post-traumatic stress disorder. Psychiatry Res 2005;140(1):27–44.

52. Menon V. Large-scale brain networks and psychopathology: a unifying triple network model. Trends Cogn Sci 2011;15(10):483–506.

53. Geuze E, Westenberg HGM, Heinecke A, et al. Thinner prefrontal cortex in veterans with posttraumatic stress disorder. Neuroimage 2008;41(3): 675–81.

54. Wrocklage KM, Averill LA, Cobb Scott J, et al. Cortical thickness reduction in combat exposed U.S. veterans with and without PTSD. Eur Neuropsychopharmacol 2017;27(5):515–25.

55. Lyoo IK, Kim JE, Yoon SJ, et al. The neurobiological role of the dorsolateral prefrontal cortex in recovery from trauma. Longitudinal brain imaging study among survivors of the South Korean subway disaster. Arch Gen Psychiatry 2011;68(7):701–13.

56. Fischl B. Automatically parcellating the human cerebral cortex. Cereb Cortex 2004;14(1):11–22.

57. Lui S, Deng W, Huang X, et al. Association of cerebral deficits with clinical symptoms in antipsychotic-naive first-episode schizophrenia: an optimized voxel-based morphometry and resting state functional connectivity study. Am J Psychiatry 2009;166(2):196–205.

58. Tregellas J. Connecting brain structure and function in schizophrenia. Am J Psychiatry 2009;166(2): 134–6.

59. Gong Q, Lui S, Sweeney JA. A selective review of cerebral abnormalities in patients with first-episode schizophrenia before and after treatment. Am J Psychiatry 2016;173(3):232–43.

60. Gusnard DA, Raichle ME, Raichle ME. Searching for a baseline: functional imaging and the resting human brain. Nat Rev Neurosci 2001;2(10):685–94.

61. Daniels JK, McFarlane AC, Bluhm RL, et al. Switching between executive and default mode networks in posttraumatic stress disorder: alterations in functional connectivity. J Psychiatry Neurosci 2010;35(4):258–66. Available at: http://www.ncbi.nlm.nih.gov/pubmed/20569651.

62. Bluhm RL, Williamson PC, Osuch EA, et al. Alterations in default network connectivity in posttraumatic stress disorder related to early-life trauma. J Psychiatry Neurosci 2009;34(3):187–94. Available at: http://www.ncbi.nlm.nih.gov/pubmed/19448848.

63. Sun Y, Wang Z, Ding W, et al. Alterations in white matter microstructure as vulnerability factors and acquired signs of traffic accident-induced PTSD. PLoS One 2013;8(12):e83473.

64. Sanjuan PM, Thoma R, Claus ED, et al. Reduced white matter integrity in the cingulum and anterior corona radiata in posttraumatic stress disorder in male combat veterans: a diffusion tensor imaging study. Psychiatry Res Neuroimaging 2013;214(3): 260–8.

65. Kennis M, van Rooij SJH, Reijnen A, et al. The predictive value of dorsal cingulate activity and fractional anisotropy on long-term PTSD symptom severity. Depress Anxiety 2017;34(5):410–8.

66. O'Doherty DCM, Ryder W, Paquola C, et al. White matter integrity alterations in post-traumatic stress disorder. Hum Brain Mapp 2018;39(3):1327–38.

67. Admon R, Leykin D, Lubin G, et al. Stress-induced reduction in hippocampal volume and connectivity with the ventromedial prefrontal cortex are related to maladaptive responses to stressful military service. Hum Brain Mapp 2013;34(11):2808–16.

68. Russman Block S, King AP, Sripada RK, et al. Behavioral and neural correlates of disrupted orienting attention in posttraumatic stress disorder. Cogn Affect Behav Neurosci 2017;17(2):422–36.

69. Sridharan D, Levitin DJ, Menon V. A critical role for the right fronto-insular cortex in switching between central-executive and default-mode networks. Proc Natl Acad Sci U S A 2008;105(34):12569–74.

70. Menon V, Uddin LQ. Saliency, switching, attention and control: a network model of insula function. Brain Struct Funct 2010;214(5–6):655–67.

71. Wolf EJ, Miller MW, Reardon AF, et al. A latent class analysis of dissociation and posttraumatic stress disorder: evidence for a dissociative subtype. Arch Gen Psychiatry 2012;69(7):698–705.

72. Lanius RA, Vermetten E, Loewenstein RJ, et al. Emotion modulation in PTSD: clinical and neurobiological evidence for a dissociative subtype. Am J Psychiatry 2010;167(6):640–7.

73. Lanius RA, Bluhm R, Lanius U, et al. A review of neuroimaging studies in PTSD: heterogeneity of

response to symptom provocation. J Psychiatr Res 2006;40(8):709–29.

74. Nicholson AA, Densmore M, Frewen PA, et al. The dissociative subtype of posttraumatic stress disorder: unique resting-state functional connectivity of basolateral and centromedial amygdala complexes. Neuropsychopharmacology 2015;40(10): 2317–26.

75. Stewart LP, White PM. Sensory filtering phenomenology in PTSD. Depress Anxiety 2008;25(1):38–45.

76. Clancy K, Ding M, Bernat E, et al. Restless "rest": intrinsic sensory hyperactivity and disinhibition in post-traumatic stress disorder. Brain 2017;140(7): 2041–50.

77. Pitman RK, Rasmusson AM, Koenen KC, et al. Biological studies of post-traumatic stress disorder. Nat Rev Neurosci 2012;13(11):769–87.

78. Kapur S, Phillips AG, Insel TR. Why has it taken so long for biological psychiatry to develop clinical tests and what to do about it? Mol Psychiatry 2012;17(12):1174–9.

79. Milham MP, Craddock RC, Klein A. Clinically useful brain imaging for neuropsychiatry: how can we get there? Depress Anxiety 2017;34(7):578–87.

80. Hoge CW, Yehuda R, Castro CA, et al. Unintended consequences of changing the definition of post-traumatic stress disorder in DSM-5: critique and call for action. JAMA Psychiatry 2016;73(7):750–2.

81. American Psychiatric Association. Diagnostic and statistical manual of mental disorders. 4th edition. Washington, DC: Text Revision; 2000.

82. Hoge CW, Riviere LA, Wilk JE, et al. The prevalence of post-traumatic stress disorder (PTSD) in US combat soldiers: a head-to-head comparison of DSM-5 versus DSM-IV-TR symptom criteria with the PTSD checklist. Lancet Psychiatry 2014;1(4):269–77.

83. Logue MW, Amstadter AB, Baker DG, et al. The Psychiatric Genomics Consortium Posttraumatic Stress Disorder Workgroup: posttraumatic stress disorder enters the age of large-scale genomic collaboration. Neuropsychopharmacology 2015;40(10):2287–97.

84. Gilbertson MW, Shenton ME, Ciszewski A, et al. Smaller hippocampal volume predicts pathologic vulnerability to psychological trauma. Nat Neurosci 2002;5(11):1242–7.

85. Schoenfeld TJ, McCausland HC, Morris HD, et al. Stress and loss of adult neurogenesis differentially reduce hippocampal volume. Biol Psychiatry 2017; 82(12):914–23.

86. Woon FL, Sood S, Hedges DW. Hippocampal volume deficits associated with exposure to psychological trauma and posttraumatic stress disorder in adults: a meta-analysis. Prog Neuropsychopharmacol Biol Psychiatry 2010;34(7):1181–8.

87. Heine VM, Maslam S, Zareno J, et al. Suppressed proliferation and apoptotic changes in the rat dentate gyrus after acute and chronic stress are reversible. Eur J Neurosci 2004;19(1):131–44. Available at: http://www.ncbi.nlm.nih.gov/pubmed/14750971.

88. Levy-Gigi E, Szabó C, Kelemen O, et al. Association among clinical response, hippocampal volume, and FKBP5 gene expression in individuals with posttraumatic stress disorder receiving cognitive behavioral therapy. Biol Psychiatry 2013;74(11):793–800.

89. Kasai K, Yamasue H, Gilbertson MW, et al. Evidence for acquired pregenual anterior cingulate gray matter loss from a twin study of combat-related post-traumatic stress disorder. Biol Psychiatry 2008; 63(6):550–6.

90. Sekiguchi A, Sugiura M, Taki Y, et al. Brain structural changes as vulnerability factors and acquired signs of post-earthquake stress. Mol Psychiatry 2013; 18(5):618–23.

91. Dahlgren MK, Laifer LM, VanElzakker MB, et al. Diminished medial prefrontal cortex activation during the recollection of stressful events is an acquired characteristic of PTSD. Psychol Med 2018;48(7): 1128–38.

92. Admon R, Milad MR, Hendler T. A causal model of post-traumatic stress disorder: disentangling predisposed from acquired neural abnormalities. Trends Cogn Sci 2013;17(7):337–47.

93. Shin LM, Bush G, Milad MR, et al. Exaggerated activation of dorsal anterior cingulate cortex during cognitive interference: a monozygotic twin study of posttraumatic stress disorder. Am J Psychiatry 2011;168(9):979–85.

94. Huang X, Gong Q, Sweeney JA, et al. Progress in psychoradiology, the clinical application of psychiatric neuroimaging. Br J Radiol 2019;92. 20181000.

95. Port JD. Diagnosis of attention deficit hyperactivity disorder by using MR imaging and radiomics: a potential tool for clinicians. Radiology 2018;287:631–2.

96. Sun H, Chen Y, Huang Q, et al. Psychoradiologic utility of MR imaging for diagnosis of attention deficit hyperactivity disorder: a radiomics analysis. Radiology 2018;287:620–30.

97. Wang D, Li M, Wang M, et al. Individual-specific functional connectivity markers track dimensional and categorical features of psychotic illness. Mol Psychiatry 2018. https://doi.org/10.1038/s41380-018-0276-1.

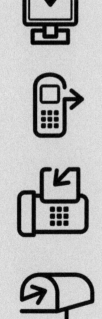

Moving?

Printed and bound by CPI Group (UK) Ltd, Croydon, CR0 4YY

03/10/2024

01040372-0009